Professional Reasoning in Healthcare

Professional Reasoning in Healthcare

Navigating Uncertainty Using the Five Finger Framework

Edited by

Helen Jeffery

Principal Lecturer, School of Occupational Therapy,
Te Pūkenga|Otago Polytechnic, New Zealand

Linda Robertson

Associate Professor Emeritus, Occupational Therapy,
Te Pūkenga, New Zealand

Jan Hendrik Roodt

Advanced Academic Facilitator, Te Pūkenga, New Zealand
Institute of Skills and Technology, New Zealand

Susan Ryan

Emerita Professor, University College Cork, Ireland

WILEY Blackwell

Registered Offices
John Wiley & Sons, Inc., 111 River Street, Hoboken, NJ 07030, USA
John Wiley & Sons Ltd, The Atrium, Southern Gate, Chichester, West Sussex, PO19 8SQ, UK

For details of our global editorial offices, customer services, and more information about Wiley products visit us at www.wiley.com.

Wiley also publishes its books in a variety of electronic formats and by print-on-demand. Some content that appears in standard print versions of this book may not be available in other formats.

Library of Congress Cataloging-in-Publication Data
Names: Jeffery, Helen (Of Otago Polytechnic) editor. | Robertson, Linda, 1947– editor. | Roodt, Jan Hendrik, editor. | Ryan, Susan (Susan Elizabeth), editor.
Title: Professional reasoning in healthcare : navigating uncertainty using the Five Finger Framework / edited by Helen Jeffery, Linda Robertson, Jan Hendrik Roodt, Susan Ryan.
Description: Hoboken, NJ : Wiley-Blackwell, 2024. | Includes bibliographical references and index.
Identifiers: LCCN 2023045745 (print) | LCCN 2023045746 (ebook) | ISBN 9781119892113 (paperback) | ISBN 9781119892151 (Adobe PDF) | ISBN 9781119892168 (epub)
Subjects: MESH: Clinical Reasoning | Clinical Decision-Making–methods. | Decision Support Techniques | Evidence-Based Medicine | Narration
Classification: LCC RA399.A1 (print) | LCC RA399.A1 (ebook) | NLM WB 142.5 | DDC 616–dc23/eng/20231108
LC record available at https://lccn.loc.gov/2023045745
LC ebook record available at https://lccn.loc.gov/2023045746

Cover Design: Wiley
Cover Images: © Sergey Ryumin/Getty Images; dTosh/Adobe Stock Photos

Set in 10.5/13pt STIXTwoText by Straive, Pondicherry, India
Printed and bound by CPI Group (UK) Ltd, Croydon, CR0 4YY

C9781119892113_090124

Contents

List of Contributors

Luciana Blaga, MOccTher. Luciana practices as an occupational therapist in New Zealand. Her experience is in acute hospital and in persistent pain. Luciana has worked in several interdisciplinary and multidisciplinary teams and maintains a focus on occupational engagement.

Sian E. Griffiths, MSc, DipCOT. Sian is a British-qualified occupational therapist with many years of practice as a therapist and educator. She has a keen interest and research background in the development of clinical/professional reasoning of occupational therapists. Sian is a principal lecturer and academic supervisor at Te Kura Whakaora Ngangahau|School of Occupational Therapy, Te Pūkenga, New Zealand.

Helen Jeffery, MOT, GCLT(7). Helen is an occupational therapist with extensive experience in community and mental health practice settings, health service management, and teaching in health and education environments. She has an interest in how therapists use theory and make decisions in practice. Her research interests are in the areas of adventure therapy and professional reasoning. Helen is a principal lecturer and academic supervisor at Te Kura Whakaora Ngangahau|Occupational Therapy School, Te Pūkenga, New Zealand.

Elizabeth Martin, PhD, GDTE, BOT(Hons), BSc (Hons). Elizabeth has practiced as an occupational therapist within orthopedic, community, and outpatient physical health. She is a senior lecturer with Te Kura Whakaora Ngangahau|Occupational Therapy School, Te Pūkenga, and researched the impact of surviving bowel cancer on occupations for her PhD study.

Kim Reay, BSc(Hons), MSc, PGCEd. Kim is a UK-trained occupational therapist and has worked in UK-based health and social services, and as an occupational therapy educator in New Zealand. Kim's interests are in exploring the meaning of evidence-based practice for learners and new practitioners, and the impact of collaborative relationships between occupational therapy and communities. Kim is a lecturer at Auckland University of Technology.

Linda Robertson, PhD has been involved in occupational therapy education for about 40 years in Scotland and New Zealand and has a special interest in professional reasoning. She has researched in the area and edited a textbook: *Clinical Reasoning in Occupational Therapy, Controversies in Practice* (2012). In 2021, Linda was awarded the NZ Order of Merit for services to occupational therapy and services to seniors.

Jan Hendrik Roodt, PhD (EngSc) (linkedin.com/in/drjanroodt) is an experienced practitioner and academic specializing in technology business establishment and management, and he contributes actively to diverse industrial and agricultural projects. Jan Hendrik also supervises postgraduate students at the New Zealand Institute of Skills and Technology, Te Pūkenga. Affiliated with professional organizations, he serves as a project and publication reviewer, as well as a journal editor.

Susan Ryan, PhD is Emerita Professor of University College Cork, Ireland. She has extensive experience in professional reasoning development and adult learning theories. She has co-authored textbooks on practice education and reasoning using narratives. She supervises qualitative research for Irish students with a focus on dementia care in Ireland.

Foreword

Dr Linda Robertson and I have had a long-distance "academic romance" for many years. It started in the 1990s when I was transitioning from being an occupational therapy and rehabilitation administrator to engaging in my doctoral work on clinical reasoning. My long-standing motivation for being in healthcare management was to support clinicians so that they in turn could provide the best care to our clients. After over twenty years in the field, I was inspired by the fascinating work of Mattingly and Fleming (1994), as their findings seemed to hold the key to a whole new understanding of how to promote effective professional reasoning and thus better practice. By then, Dr Robertson was already engaged in academics and following the same work. She, along with several of her colleagues, continued to advance our understanding of what we now call professional reasoning. I am so pleased they joined to offer this new text: *Professional Reasoning in Healthcare: Navigating Uncertainty using the Five Finger Framework* edited by Jeffery, Roodt, Robertson, and Ryan. I am honored to introduce this important new contribution, as they make the leap from *understanding* professional reasoning to *improving* professional reasoning.

My overriding emotion while reading this new text is one of gratitude. So let me start by saying thank you. Thanks for synthesizing the many things we know about professional reasoning into a very practical and digestible resource. Thanks for working with the complexity to offer real, concrete, and doable approaches for improving professional reasoning. Thanks for making your suggestions both profound and easy to read. Thanks for using real stories of real practitioners to show how this works in practice. Thanks for broadening the views on client and culture. Thanks for opening new horizons for research to improve practice. In short, thanks for "handing us" the five-finger framework. It will work for students, it will work for practitioners, it will work for educators, and it will work for scholars. Well done.

Barbara A. Boyt Schell, PhD, OT, FAOTA

Professor Emeritus, School of Occupational Therapy, Brenau University Co-owner, Schell Consulting

REFERENCE

Mattingly, C., & Fleming, M. H. (1994). *Clinical reasoning – forms of inquiry in a therapeutic practice*. F.A. Davis.

Preface

This book, written for practitioners, students, and educators, is a response to changes in society's expectations of health professionals and the impact on delivery of services. Traditionally, specialization was the hallmark of the expert. However, in the current world of complex practice, professionals require systems-level thinking where it is the generalist who becomes the "artful master." In order to thrive in a world that demands constant change where there is not necessarily a right or wrong answer (the so-called "wicked" problems), strong frameworks are needed for decision making.

In response to this acknowledged threat to "practice as usual," a framework has been developed that will impact on reasoning and assist professionals to work effectively in the current working environment. This has been named the Five Finger Framework (FFF) and provides a simple structure to guide complex thinking. Essentially, it encourages the use of evidence from a diverse range of sources to inform decisions and stimulates a questioning approach. It uses the metaphor of the hand to stimulate complicated critical thinking: the fingers trigger the reader to explore research-based literature, the environment where the practice is situated, the client/family, the expertise of others, and what is integral to the self. The FFF has the potential to stimulate habitual scrutiny of multiple sources of information and viewpoints in a straightforward way to provide an awareness of the problem solver's situation. From this awareness, anticipatory thinking

can be encouraged to ensure that a range of possible contributory factors are considered and helpful solutions generated. The FFF provides a structure that enhances both the visibility and traceability of thinking.

This book is written using narratives – each of the fingers on the framework is portrayed in a chapter written in the first person as a story from the perspective of a health practitioner. Story telling enables natural engagement with content and enhances focus on and motivation for the reading. The stories provide the reader with a way to imagine the situation and the professional reasoning that is informing the practitioner's response. Importantly, the nonlinear reality of professional reasoning processes and the messiness of everyday practice are illustrated. Despite the narrative nature of the writing style making the chapters potentially an "easy read," theory is integrated and the complexity integral to reasoning processes and decision making is made evident. The writing style further enhances the visibility of thinking provided in the Five Finger Framework.

Both the FFF itself and how it is described, justified, and illustrated in this text are fundamentally based on the concept of situated learning. This learning theory follows a premise that knowledge and resultant action are uniquely formed by individuals in direct response to their situation, environment, and the people they interact with. Each of the chapters related to the fingers brings to life how learning is situated, and the power of reflexivity in deepening and strengthening the impact of learning.

For readers looking for the rigorous underpinnings of the work, the theoretical and practical motivators for the FFF are covered in some detail in Chapter 2. The situated and reflexive practice in fields spanning several disciplines is discussed with a focus on reflective thinking skills, transformative learning, and sense making. Chapter 8 covers the increasing need for transdisciplinary thinking in these fields and introduces a complexity-based view on ethics and values. The final chapter contains tools and tips for using this book in practice and in an educational setting.

Acknowledgments

Our belief is that professional reasoning is fundamental to the quality of health service provision. This contribution to literature in professional reasoning is the culmination of effort on the part of many. It represents not only our own research, but a drawing from and synthesis of theory and discourse from other academics. We commend and are grateful for all who are working on advancing healthcare practice through deepening and sharing knowledge of professional reasoning.

We would like to acknowledge the willing sharing of ideas, opinions, and practices from clinicians, lecturers, and students in our own research. The basis of the Five Finger Framework emerged from those discussions and interviews – thank you for your insights and openness.

Writing in a style that is relaxed and accessible but also portrays complex theories and processes is challenging. We are grateful to the many people from diverse professions and practice areas who were prepared to read chapters through a particular lens. These included Indigenous practitioners and academics, and those from the disciplines of speech and language therapy, physiotherapy, social work, counseling, and occupational therapy. We also thank Dr Sheena Blair (occupational therapist) whose deep knowledge and sharp mind helped us tighten and tidy the work and reassured us of its value. Special thanks is also due to Professor Barbara Schell for her willingness to immerse herself in the manuscript and write a foreword for the text.

Finally, we acknowledge you, the reader of this text, whether you are an educator, student, practitioner, or manager. Your preparedness to read and ponder how a professional reasoning framework such as this might influence your work and ultimately enhance the outcomes for the people who access your services is commendable.

Helen Jeffery, Linda Robertson,
Jan Hendrik Roodt, Susan Ryan

Praise for *Professional Reasoning in Healthcare: Navigating Uncertainty Using the Five Finger Framework*

An essential tool and a great insight to the decision-making skills that health professionals go through on a daily basis – a must-read for all practitioners, new, and seasoned!
Lara Gallichan, BSc(Hons), Speech and Language Therapist, NZSTA

Written in a clear and accessible manner, there is no doubt this book will be an invaluable resource for students, clinicians, and teachers alike. By providing real-world examples, the reader easily appreciates the value of the Five Finger Framework and how it can improve their professional reasoning and practice. This book should be compulsory reading for all students, and I would highly recommend it to all practicing healthcare workers.
Dr Ruth Jeffery, PhD, MSc, PGDip Med Rad Sci(NM), LLB(Hons), BA, BSc, NZDMI

The ability to critically reflect upon the way that professional reasoning and judgment occurs is pivotal and is profoundly ethical for practice, research, and leadership. Amongst the unique features of this text is the introduction of the Five Finger Framework to assist lifelong learners to comprehensively problem pose and problem solve. This resonates well with situated learning with its focus upon context, interpersonal relationships, and shared decision making.
    The book is culturally aware, transdisciplinary, and has the potential to become a core text for learners at all levels of education, particularly for those within practice-based education and mentorship relationships.
Dr Sheena E.E. Blair, DipOT, MEd, ED, FRCOT

Thanks for offering real, concrete, and doable approaches for improving professional reasoning, using real stories of real practitioners to show how this works in practice, broadening the views on client and culture. In short, thanks for "handing us" the Five Finger Framework. It will work for students, practitioners, educators, and scholars. I would adopt it in a heartbeat if I were still teaching!
Barbara A. Schell, Professor Emerita, School of Occupational Therapy, Brenau University, PhD, OT/L, FAOTA

This internationally relevant text presents the Five Finger Framework as a tool for enabling practice reasoning, critical reflection, and decision making across a range of transdisciplinary approaches in health and social care settings. The metaphor of a hand unfolds a structured process for thinking through many-layered aspects to reach the end goal we all aim for – working effectively, visibly and in a traceable and thus accountable manner for collaborative solution-focused approaches.
Margaret McKenzie, Associate Professor, Registered Social Worker (NZ)

CHAPTER 1

Synthesizing Knowledge for Situated Practice: The Five Finger Framework

Historical Influences on Professional Reasoning

Helen Jeffery[1] and Susan Ryan[2]

[1]*Principal Lecturer, School of Occupational Therapy, Te Pūkenga|Otago Polytechnic, New Zealand*
[2]*Emerita Professor, University College Cork, Ireland*

INTRODUCTION

Professional reasoning is the thinking that sits behind practice decisions. It informs what we do and how we do it, and is influenced by who we are, where we are and what we know, believe, and value. How we reason in practice depends on the knowledge networks that we develop as we practice. Experienced clinicians have difficulty explaining their reasoning because it is based on their own experiences and stored in an idiosyncratic way. The task for the novice is to develop their own knowledge base as they practice and to organize this so that it makes sense to them and can be recalled as needed. Learning from experience is an ongoing process which can be enhanced by ensuring the learner has opportunities to recall learning experiences and to make sense of them. Frameworks that provide guidelines for reflection can assist the learner to have a greater awareness of potential influences on their actions.

This textbook presents the Five Finger Framework as a metaphor that identifies and integrates elements of reasoning (see Figure 1.1). The framework was developed following research conducted by lecturers in occupational therapy education (Jeffery et al., 2021). The aim was to better prepare occupational therapy students to be effective evidence-based practitioners by identifying strategies that could be used in the curriculum to hone professional reasoning skills.

Professional Reasoning in Healthcare: Navigating Uncertainty Using the Five Finger Framework, First Edition.
Edited by Helen Jeffery, Linda Robertson, Jan Hendrik Roodt, and Susan Ryan.
© 2024 John Wiley & Sons Ltd. Published 2024 by John Wiley & Sons Ltd.

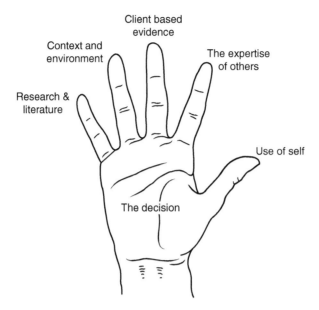

FIGURE 1.1   The Five Finger Framework.

The Five Finger Framework draws together the key elements that inform professional reasoning. Depicted as a hand, with the decision to be made or the problem to be solved in the palm of the hand, the framework provides an easy-to-remember structure that enables reasoning that is both broad and deep. The comprehensiveness of decision making can be made visible and therefore be shared with and used by learners and facilitators of learning both in education and in practice. Additionally, the framework enables the development of habits and strategies that promote considered professional reasoning throughout the practitioner's career (Benfield & Jeffery, 2022).

Each of the five fingers represents an essential source of information and evidence to inform professional decision making. The palm of the hand holds the decision or problem posed, i.e., about what you will do, what you are doing or what you did do. The thumb, representing the self (you), touches base with each of the other fingers as the situation is worked through. The

sources of evidence to inform professional decision making represented by the fingers of the hand are as follows.

1. **Research and literature:** from policy, published research, textbooks and reports, practice models and theories, foundational knowledge of the profession – practice decisions that are based on academic rigor.

2. **Context and environment:** include the workplace culture, systems and resources, the local community culture and resources, protocols, and procedures – practice decisions that reflect local best practice.

3. **Client:** collaboration with client, client's knowledge and expertise, families and carers' perspective and situation – practice decisions that are right for the client.

4. **Expertise of others:** informed by local practitioners with helpful knowledge through to international experts, accessed through conversations, conferences, and internet

resources – practice decisions are in part informed by knowledge-able others.

5. **Use of self:** the knowledge held by the practitioner in conjunction with the therapeutic use of self, relationship-building skills, self-awareness, reflective practice, and awareness of one's own culture – practice decision that are right for you.

This introductory chapter is in three parts. *Part One* provides some historical context to set the scene in terms of the development of professions and the introduction of professional reasoning. An overview of the history of the growth of health professions related to knowledge generation is presented to provide context for the complexities experienced in professional reasoning today. *Part Two* describes some of the external influences that need to be taken into consideration when working through reasoning in practice. This includes changes internationally in healthcare provision and growing awareness of cultural safety, two of many factors that influence professional reasoning processes and practices. These are linked to and provide justification for the development of the elements in the Five Finger Framework. *Part Three* gives a brief overview of subsequent chapters.

PART ONE: HISTORICAL PERSPECTIVES

This section provides an overview of the important historical factors in the development of healthcare that have influenced professionals' thinking and practice. Most contemporary health professions date back to their commencement in the nineteenth or early twentieth centuries. Over time, each has altered profoundly as new knowledge is generated through science and research, and as society has changed. New knowledge is synthesized into existing bodies of knowledge (Higgs & Edwards, 1999) and both strengthens some knowledge and makes some obsolete. This synthesis of diverse knowledge creates innovative practices within professions, as new theory is used as a stepping stone to expand professional boundaries. So, keeping in mind these constant changes, professions should be thought of as being fluid entities within their own lifecycles (Dower et al., 2001). They have constantly evolved, developed, and changed through the decades as they are exposed to influences within and outside the profession, and will continue to do so.

Professionalization

To become a health professional involves long periods of theoretical and practical training resulting in a formal qualification (Dower et al., 2001). Although many professions have a world body or organization charged with maintaining international professional standards, their work is bound by understanding that what works in one country may not work in another – context of practice and cultural mores are powerful influences on practice. The understanding a practitioner has of their professional scope and responsibilities, the nature of their professional identity, and the context they are situated in all form a basis for their professional decision making.

The profession that a person is a part of will contribute to determine what practice decisions are made, e.g., an occupational therapist will view a particular client through a different lens from a nurse, physiotherapist, or social worker, and have very different assessments and intervention parameters to work within. However, decisions are also influenced by who the practitioner is and the relationship they hold with the client – professional identity is broader than the parameters of the profession itself.

As professions have widened and deepened their knowledge base and practices, work has become more complex and multilayered. Of note is the concept of specialization – the increase in what can be known creates space for increasing numbers of specialist people and services, consequentially compartmentalizing the work within professions and the experience of the client (Skinner et al., 2015). Even professions that are philosophically grounded in holistic practice offer specialist services, for example occupational therapists in the role of hand therapist. Conversely, practice settings are also becoming more diverse in what they offer and many new fields, specialties, and services are being promoted and developed (Skinner et al., 2015). In many settings, the pace of healthcare practice has accelerated, and specialist service is expected, with increased demands placed on early career practitioners to work at higher levels of knowledge and responsibility and at a faster pace. Health professionals now, more than ever, need to be able to remain current in their evidence base for practice, be responsive to change and prepared to handle the dissonance that is often apparent between specialist practice and client-centered holistic healthcare.

Professional Reasoning

Exploration of professional reasoning processes and practices has been evident in health literature over recent decades and has resulted in the development of theories and models to explain, teach, and guide the processes that enable safe decision making in health practice. This has its roots in part in North American and Canadian medical educators (Cranton, 1983; Eisner, 1979). These academics introduced different learning and assessment methods to examine the thinking and reasoning of their medical students to encourage them to be more systematic and scientific. After that introductory work, other professions followed suit.

In the mid-1980s, the American Occupational Therapy Association (AOTA) employed an anthropologist, Dr Cheryl Mattingly (1991), to study the reasoning of a group of occupational therapists. Coming from a different discipline entirely, she used a "bottom-up" grounded approach to this study which was different from the analytical and comparative methods the medical educators used. She employed qualitative research methods and gathered narratives and stories to explore the decision making of therapists. Her work was later complemented by an occupational therapy educator, Fleming, who analyzed and presented Mattingly's work in the form of different tracks – procedural, interactive, and conditional, each focusing on a different aspect of professional reasoning (Fleming, 1991; Mattingly & Fleming, 1994).

PART TWO: INFLUENCES ON REASONING

This section focuses on some of the recent changes in society, foundational knowledge, and contexts of health practices that have influenced professional reasoning in the five areas that form the Five Finger Framework.

Influences of "Self" on Reasoning

All professional decisions are centered to a greater or lesser degree in the "self" – who we are, our culture, our knowledge, skills, and attitudes all impact the decisions we make. However, our ways of knowing are developed from personal experiences of practice and include technical, practical, social, political, and economic knowledge as well as self-knowledge (Kinsella, 2001). Some of our knowledge is explicit and can clearly be identified while other knowledge is implicit and is difficult to explain to others but is evident in our actions. "Reflective approaches suggest that it is important to examine our actions in practice in order to discover this implicit knowledge which influences what we actually do in practice" (Kinsella, 2001, p. 196).

In the 1980s, Professor Donald Schön, a North American educator, developed an influential framework for reflection (Schön, 1983). The framework was intended for learners to reflect on their ideas retrospectively, having made decisions or completed piece of work, to recognize potential improvements to their practice. In Australia, Boud et al. (1985) also designed a model of reflection consisting of three parts whereby a learner/practitioner reflected on their ideas before, during, and after an event to encourage intentional thinking about what they might do (prospective), what they are doing (in the moment), and what they did do (retrospective). Subsequently, many models to guide reflection have been developed, and for many people, being reflective has become habitual. It is now often advocated in professional practice as a way of enabling practitioners to develop a critical understanding of their own practice.

There is more to the personal influence on reasoning than the capacity to reflect. Practitioners require self-awareness of their skills, attitudes, knowledge, and their own culture, including their cultural biases (both conscious and unconscious). How they understand the world around them and the perspectives they hold influence the decisions they come to. Practitioners therefore have an ethical responsibility to maintain awareness of and pay attention to their own perspective in any situation. Being able to recognize, acknowledge, and

consider this positionality, the influence it has on the decisions we make and the potential influence on clients' decisions is important (Delany et al., 2010). Additionally, the capacity to hear and respond to feedback, to form, maintain, and repair therapeutic relationships, and to develop practice that is aligned with personal values are all influences on practice decisions.

The Influence of the Expertise of Others on Reasoning

An integral element of professional reasoning and influence on professional decisions is know-how shared with us and recommendations made by others who are more knowledgeable or experienced than we are (Wieringa & Greenhalgh, 2015). We create and refine ways of viewing our world, based in part on the opinions of colleagues and experts and our agreement and consensus with them.

One way to make use of new knowledge is through direct contact with local and international experts – seeing and hearing ideas to augment reading articles enhances understanding. The internet and modern communication platforms have enabled the capacity for rapid dissemination of knowledge and research findings in this way. It is not just newly published knowledge but also access to those holding expertise that is now readily available. For instance, the availability of recorded presentations, online discussions, online conferences, and a variety of web-based presentations make learning from this expertise accessible and affordable for most. These opportunities enhance the capacity to connect with and learn from developments in our respective professional fields across different nations.

Internet-based communication has developed through platforms and applications which make it easier to connect directly with knowledgeable others and to engage directly with them – a practice that is becoming normalized. This access is, of course, open to the world – we not only have the capacity to explore knowledge from our own discipline but also from others, borrow from theory, merge concepts, and deepen understanding of each other and the work we do. This is immensely helpful in this era of interdisciplinary work, where in many practice areas there is more blurring of professional boundaries than in the past. In contrast to specialization, there is also a trend toward more generic work within specialist teams.

A challenge can be for practitioners to rationalize their profession-specific reasoning to maintain professional identity in a close work environment where there is a tendency to merge roles (Best & Williams, 2019).

Influences of the Client on Reasoning

The professional's relationship with a client has shifted over time as professionals have gained greater awareness of the importance of knowing the overall client's needs and the value of working in collaboration with that client. This movement toward a collaborative approach with the client was first emphasized in the work of psychologist Carl Rogers (1951) who founded the humanistic approach to healthcare. The overall movement seen in this approach is from a place where the client seeks intervention from an expert practitioner to a place where they can work alongside a practitioner to achieve their goals. It is now crucial that the notion of "one size fits all" is not followed and that personalized practice is enhanced as much as is reasonably possible (Dower et al., 2001).

The advent of the internet also facilitated a profound change in the place clients have in their healthcare. Represented on the Five Finger Framework as the client finger,

the people we work with now have easy access to information. Consequently, the level of health/knowledge literacy in many populations has increased exponentially. People are becoming more articulate and more educated and may be more demanding of better professional services. Clients may now have more specific expectations of health professionals and be more informed of their options in terms of service. There is more openness and discussion in the media, highly developed internet-based communication platforms that support client-led support groups, discussion forums, and shared problem-solving avenues for clients. This access to knowledge and education by everyone is one of many drivers toward client empowerment and involvement in practice decisions.

As clients are empowered to voice their opinions, and professionals are no longer seen as the fount of all knowledge, collaboration in joint professional decision making is enabled. The client voice is also evident in the increase of value and recognition placed on qualitative research. Its use of stories, narratives, and interviews over the more scientific research has added to the knowledge base around client experiences, and what works and does not work for them. This has in turn led to their involvement not just in their own healthcare decisions but in service development, monitoring of and advising on quality of services, and input into legislation. Clients are more able to voice their perspective so the challenge is for practitioners to hear this and to ensure their professional reasoning processes are made in collaboration with the client.

Context – Influence of Resources and Culture on Reasoning

The knowledge explosion has had a profound impact on what is possible in professional practice, with resultant challenges related to access, equity, and affordability. An individual's access to best practice is dependent on where they live, the health structures in their country and local community, and the management of financial and other resources. Management structures and resultant decisions in many countries now revolve more around finances than care, and efficiencies must take precedence. Managers have tight budgets to administer whilst having greater diversity in products to fund, services to include, and specialists to employ, as well as other demands from practitioners and clients. Managerial decisions impact the number of staff employed, the model of service provision used, and, importantly, the amount of time available for intervention, as well as the environments in which intervention can occur. For many practitioners, professional reasoning is influenced by their compliance with organizational management requirements, and "decisions are made to meet the demands of work and where the individual is a cog in the machine" (Fish & de Cossart, 2019, p. 102). These demands, which include workflow, work structure, and access to material and human resources, influence professional reasoning on a day-to-day basis.

People have, of course, traveled throughout history but more so in recent centuries and dramatically so in recent decades, and globalization has become a norm. As health beliefs and values are culturally bound, the cultural influence on professional reasoning is of paramount importance. A significant population movement in previous centuries was through colonization of countries with established Indigenous populations. Those countries colonized in more recent history are now grappling with the challenges associated with the resultant health, social, and political wellbeing of their Indigenous people and the systemic racism that developed through the dominance of the colonizing culture (McIntosh et al., 2021). In these countries, there is now a growing call for past wrongs to be put right, for enablement of Indigenous power and autonomy, for restoration of Indigenous language and traditions and, importantly, equity in health outcomes. An integral part of choices regarding professional decisions is whether the client is Indigenous and how connected they are to their culture. Although there are a growing number of Indigenous health providers, in a large proportion of these countries services are provided by the still dominant culture through a Eurocentric lens. "A single western scientific model of the world is no longer the only acceptable model of reality" (Dower et al., 2001, p. 2). Intentional consideration of this influences who the service providers should be, what intervention is appropriate, and where and how it can be implemented.

Air travel has exponentially increased speed of communication and the ability to travel long distances quickly and affordably. The era of globalization has a significant impact on how health services are delivered in many countries. It is not unusual for practitioners to work across countries or to migrate to help fill professional shortages in other parts of the world, or for patients to travel for surgery, medical intervention, or other services. Immediate access to current affairs enables people to appreciate what is happening on an international level, which in turn promotes population movement. We now see people moving to other countries for a plethora of reasons, including job opportunities, political or economic reasons, fundamental safety reasons or simply to experience different cultures and climates.

Again, this may not seem important in terms of professional reasoning, but practitioners are increasingly working in multicultural societies, where some groups are marginalized, some have significant trauma histories, and many are estranged from families and usual supports. Coupled with developing understanding of the link between personal history, culture, and health, practitioners are now likely to meet with clients whose enculturated views and beliefs may conflict with their own (Wasserman & Loftus, 2019).

In addition to the above, practitioners themselves may relocate – it is not unusual to practice in a population that has vastly different cultural norms from the practitioner's own. The capacity for cultural awareness, sensitivity, and safety is paramount in day-to-day practice in many communities and services. Factors in globalization are illustrated in Figure 1.2.

Influence of Knowledge and Research on Reasoning

One of the main identifiers and boundaries of a profession is the research knowledge the members draw from and develop. In the early days of the twentieth century, many of the newer health professions engaged in little research. Health professional education

opportunities began "on the floor" as they engaged in situated learning. This practical and contextualized learning then developed into more formal education in technical colleges and then universities where research methods became part of the higher-level program. Degree status was awarded for many health professions in the 1980s and 1990s, and only then did they include some forms of research-based education. In health science curricula, the use of published research, learning about research, participation in ongoing research studies, and conducting research in practice was a phenomenon derived from this period. Originally used to inform population health on a broad scale, the expectation is now to base individual practice decisions on research evidence, whether it be quantitative or qualitative methods (Lambert, 2006).

Prior to research-based decisions, many practice decisions were based on what the practitioner understood, believed, had tried, or had seen others do (Lambert, 2006). This resulted in some important practice

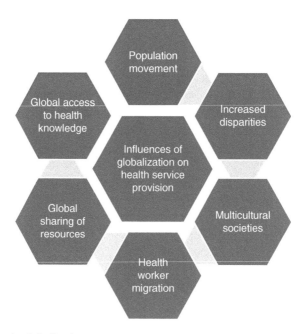

FIGURE 1.2   Factors in globalization.

development but, unfortunately, some practitioners applied treatments that were unsafe, ineffective, or not suited to a particular population. These less informed practices were challenged in 1991 by a Canadian physician, Dr Gordon Guyatt, who wanted to shift the emphasis in clinical decision making from intuition and unsystematic clinical experience to scientific, clinically relevant research that provided evidence of efficacy (Guyatt et al., 1992). This was reinforced by the work of Sackett (Lambert, 2006; Thoma & Eaves, 2015), and heralded the era of evidence-based medicine. This mantle was then adopted by other health professions in the form of evidence-based practice (Taylor, 2000).

Professional education, including health, has now reached doctoral level and the amount of postdoctoral research being conducted has increased exponentially. The resultant surge in knowledge generation has dramatically changed service provision from government level down to individual practitioners through these research findings as they inform services at all levels. The use of research to develop, enhance, and inform practice is now an expectation. Evidence-based practice processes must now be integral to our professional reasoning.

The generation of research knowledge of itself is highly influential on professional decision making. However, the advent of the internet and the subsequent ability to disseminate research findings has created a knowledge explosion that is easy to access yet difficult to keep on top of. This has created a challenge for beginning practitioners, who search for certainty and concrete answers in environments where there is ambiguity. Often termed as VUCA (Volatility, Uncertainty, Complexity, Ambiguity) (Pandit, 2020), the pace of change in today's world is difficult to manage for practitioners who crave stability, certainty,

and clarity. But, as a practicing professional in this electronic era, being comfortable with uncertainty is important. With such a plethora of online research articles available on the internet, the current health practitioner requires skills in finding and selecting what is most useful. This dilemma of choice is vastly different from previous learning methods when students learned the content from a textbook or purely from their tutors or peers as historically was the norm.

Research requires contextualization and translation to fit the specific situation, and in isolation often does not provide adequate evidence to make good practice decisions. One element of contextualization is ensuring that the research selected is reviewed through a critical lens in terms of trustworthiness and utility. The diverse knowledges need to be synthesized to create understanding that is contextually relevant and useful for practice. Furthermore, some research results that match and work in one culture may not be suitable for another – findings may need to be contextualized to meet the needs of the population. For many professions, there are diverse options emerging in terms of assessment and intervention or practice. The amount of choice can be overwhelming and requires in-depth discussions and wider reasoning before decisions are made. Health professionals need to look both within and beyond the literature available to them for support in making professional decisions. Ideally, the practice environment is set up in a way that enables pragmatic access to appropriate research through knowledge translation and practice guidelines.

In summary, this chapter provides background to illustrate the complexity of practice decisions at this point in history and links the factors to the Five Finger Framework. This flexible framework will guide inquiry and enable both learners and practitioners to create optimal and evidence-based practice decisions that are appropriate for themselves, their clients, and their context (Jeffery et al., 2021). The framework is designed to assist learners and practitioners to operate in diverse practice environments and is responsive to the ongoing critique that has accompanied the evidence-based practice movement, and to ongoing changes in healthcare provision.

PART THREE: OVERVIEW OF THE CHAPTERS

The reader has been introduced to some of the most important influences on professional development in the past two centuries culminating in the current times. This has provided a rationale for the development of The Five Finger Framework.

The ongoing chapters in this text have been designed to illustrate each section of this framework in depth through practice--based narratives. Below is an overview of the contents.

Chapter 2: The Five Finger Framework: Development and Rationale

Fostering Thinking Skills

This chapter will report on the findings of the study that informed the development of a flexible "thinking" framework that encourages both a broad and critical exploration of elements of occupational therapy reasoning for practice. A broadening of essential features of being evidence based is included, asking relevant questions and intentional exploration of the self and others in the local context. The framework promotes the use of the metaphor of the hand with each of the five fingers representing the elements that are essential to

consider when making decisions in practice. While it is often said that professional reasoning is more than using research evidence, there is little clarity in the literature about the other components and even less attention paid to how these are integrated into decision making and student learning. This chapter makes these aspects explicit by providing transparency around the components that are integrated into decision making. Using recent research, it will also postulate a stance on different positions taken that indicate expertise and how these impact on professional development.

> ### Key Points
> - Skills of being a critical thinker
> - Use of metaphor in learning
> - From evidence-based practice to local best practice
> - Introduction of the Five Finger Framework

Chapter 3: Grasping the Whole: The Practitioner Perspective

Practitioner Influences on Professional Decisions

The way knowledge is constructed is profoundly influenced by how we handle information, interactions, and experiences to enable a fit with who we are and what we already know, believe, and value. Self-awareness or holding an understanding of who we are and how we practice enhances our capacity to integrate new knowledge and skills. Integral to this is also the ability to reflect both prospectively (what might we do) and retrospectively (what did we do), and to use insights gained through reflective processes to effect changes in reasoning or practice. Awareness of personal cultural influences and biases promotes cultural sensitivity and enhances capacity to form therapeutic relationships. Conscious use of self as a tool in therapy is enabled through integration of who we are, what is important to us, what we know, and what we know how to do. Learning from others is in part dependent on ability to hear and respond to feedback. Capacity to maintain competence to continue to develop professionally is reliant on preparedness to touch base with each of the other fingers, and to integrate learning into our professional self. The voice in the chapter is that of an occupational therapist.

> **Key Points**
>
> - Threshold concepts
> - Self-awareness
> - Conscious and unconscious bias
> - Reflective practice
> - Therapeutic use of self

Chapter 4: Using the Expertise of Others: Many Hands Make Light Work

Accessing Knowledge from Others to Inform Professional Decisions

Tapping into the knowledge that others hold to augment what we already know provides reassurance and enables development of knowledge and skills. Social learning theory informs understanding of the value and processes behind learning from others. Learning occurs through listening to, observing, conversing with, and questioning others. Strategies to intentionally select and use the expertise of others are useful and can be facilitated directly and indirectly. Direct access to the expertise of others is facilitated through supervision, colleagues, and peers to ask questions of, along with opportunities for further education such as attendance at

conferences and use of internet resources. The expertise of others is available indirectly through managerial systems that support intentional knowledge translation and strategies for this to flow through to assessment and intervention processes. Importantly, peer learning theory that utilizes a constructivist approach to learning supports the value of intentional peer-led groups, peer supervision, and involvement in communities of practice. The voice in the chapter is that of a physiotherapist.

> **Key Points**
>
> - Accessing expertise
> - Social learning theory
> - Communities of practice
> - Knowledge translation
> - Peer learning

Chapter 5: Walking Hand in Hand: Collaborative Practice

Eliciting and Incorporating Client Perspectives

Person-centered practice comes from a humanistic perspective and focuses on the premise that the client is central to intervention and in an equal relationship with the therapist. Genuine person-centered practice is reliant on the therapist being able to appreciate the client's position and perspective, to utilize the expertise the client brings of their situation to positive effect, and to be culturally safe in their practice. Person-centered practice is evident not just in the relationship between therapist and client, but also in interventions the therapist intentionally selects to enhance the client's capacity to work in partnership, and in background structures and processes that enable this way of working for the therapist. These include feedback-informed processes and client education to enhance informed decisions. Although the term "person or client centeredness" intimates an individual, this approach is equally important when working with families, groups or communities. What the client brings to the therapy process and how they work together with the therapist profoundly influence the decisions made by the therapist on a day-to-day basis. The voice in the chapter is that of a speech and language therapist.

> ## Key Points
>
> - Who is the client?
> - Client as expert
> - Power and relationship
> - Facilitating collaboration
> - Feedback-informed intervention

Chapter 6: Knowing the Context like the Back of Your Hand

Contextual Influences on Professional Reasoning

This chapter will encourage the development of an understanding of the environment's impact on practice. Much of this is not well understood by practitioners and this chapter will encourage identification of the structures and protocols that impact on practice. Importantly, the broader environment can profoundly influence practice decisions but is rarely considered in intentional reasoning processes. The culture of the local community (ethnicity, urban or rural, lower or higher socioeconomic status, and educational levels, among other factors) has implications for the client base as well as for professional reasoning processes. Equally important is an understanding of the practice setting. The culture of the team, the workflow processes and structure, and the resources available all

influence professional reasoning and impact on practice decisions. The voice in the chapter is that of a social worker.

> ## Key Points
>
> - Team culture
> - Practice setting guidelines, systems, and processes
> - Resources in practice setting and in wider community
> - Local culture
> - Identifying local best practice
> - How practice is shaped by the context

Chapter 7: Letting the Research Lend a Hand

Evaluating, Synthesizing, and Implementing Knowledges

This chapter will review the current understanding of how literature and research can be used as valid sources of evidence. Enablers and barriers to the use of literature to inform practice will be discussed, and strategies to enhance the use of literature in practice presented. Ideas and resources will be provided to enable critical review of the quality of the literature. To complement formal research, current textbooks will be endorsed as important sources of understandings of practice that not only record "good" practice but also identify key authors in particular fields of practice. Additionally, models and frameworks that structure the implementation of research into practice are endorsed, and their use as tools within practice is encouraged. Shortcuts to locating reviews of research relevant to specific practice areas will be explored and promoted as valuable resources and good use of time. Ideas will be provided to assist the integration of research evidence into practice. The integration of knowledge from a mix of disciplines into practice will also be discussed. The voice in the chapter is that of an interprofessional team.

Key Points

- Critical view of the choice of research, literature, and theory
- Asking questions of the literature
- Practical strategies for use of literature conducive to busy, thoughtful practice
- The mobile mind – being intentional and selective with research evidence
- Barriers and enablers to using research evidence in practice

---

Chapter 8: Synthesizing World Views

Transdisciplinarity and the Five Finger Framework

The wisdom that health practitioners draw on every day includes a wide range of disciplines and world views. Occupational therapy is one such profession, where a key approach is that of pragmatic problem solving. Like some of the other multidisciplinary vocations, including system design engineering, information technology practitioners and those in multi-resource agriculture, the question of who we are and what we do is not easy to answer. Nor is it easy to manage the uncertainty and risks inherent to practicing in a field with such a broad scope. This chapter covers the concept of transdisciplinarity, working within, across and beyond the traditional disciplines, as a way of explaining what practitioners do,

how they do it, and how they make decisions under uncertainty. We use the profession of occupational therapy to illustrate some points, but this chapter is neither solely about nor for occupational therapists alone. The ethical imperative is included in the discussion as a moral position, a "Values North Star." It opens a way of acting and doing in a manner that potentially grounds work in a deeper respectful, responsible foundation and points to shifts in how one approaches the education of future practitioners.

Key Points

- Awareness of diverse worldviews
- Origins of transdisciplinarity
- Philosophical positions and theory focused on action
- A transdisciplinary value system and ethical imperative
- Using the Five Finger Framework in a transdisciplinary context

---

Chapter 9: Tools for Implementing the Five Finger Framework

Ideas, Activities, and Tips for Practice and Education Settings

Frameworks provide a way of putting synthesized knowledge into practice – whether the "practice" be thinking or action. This chapter offers some tools and activity ideas that can be used by individuals or groups using the Five Finger Framework. The tools provide some structure to use of the framework in specific situations, and some creativity in how learners and practitioners might integrate its use into their work. Most of the tools are useful for learners in educational settings, novice practitioners, and experienced practitioners.

REFERENCES

Benfield, A., & Jeffery, H. (2022). Exploring evidence-based practice implementation by occupational therapists: implications for fieldwork. *Journal of Occupational Therapy Education*, *6*(4), 10–20.

Best, S., & Williams, S. (2019). Professional identity in interprofessional teams: findings from a scoping review. *Journal of Interprofessional Care*, *33*(2), 170–181.

Boud, D., Keogh, R., & Walker, D. (1985). Promoting reflection in learning: a model. In D. Boud, R. Keogh, & D. Walker (Eds.), *Reflection: Turning experience into learning* (pp. 18–40). Kogan Page.

Cranton, P. (1983). Transfer of student learning in medical education. *Journal of Medical Education*, *58*(2), 126–135.

Delany, C. M., Edwards, I., Jensen, G. M., & Skinner, E. (2010). Closing the gap between ethics knowledge and practice through active engagement: an applied model of physical therapy ethics. *Physical Therapy*, *90*(7), 1068–1078.

Dower, C., O'Neil, E. H., & Hough, H. J. (2001). *Profiling the professions: A model for evaluating emerging health professions.* Center for the Health Professions, University of California, San Francisco.

Eisner, E. (1979). *The educational imagination: On design and evaluation of school programs*. Macmillan Publishing.

Fish, D., & de Cossart, L. (2019). Clinical thinking, client expectations and patient-centred care. In J. Higgs, G. M. Jensen, S. Loftus, & N. Christensen (Eds.), *Clinical reasoning in health professions* (pp. 97–108). Elsevier.

Fleming, M. H. (1991). The therapist with the three-track mind. *American Journal of Occupational Therapy*, *45*(11), 1007–1014.

Guyatt, G., Cairns, J., Churchill, D., Cook, D., Haynes, B., Hirsh, J., & Tugwell, P. (1992). Evidence-based medicine: a new approach to teaching the practice of medicine. *JAMA*, *268*(17), 2420–2425.

Higgs, J., & Edwards, H. (1999). Educating beginning practitioners in the health professions. In J. Higgs & H. Edwards (Eds.), *Educating beginning practitioners: Challenges for health professional education* (pp. 3–9). Butterworth-Heinemann.

Jeffrey, H., Robertson, L., & Reay, K. (2021). Sources of evidence for professional decision-making in novice occupational therapy practitioners: clinicians' perspectives. *British Journal of Occupational Therapy*, *84*(6), 346–354.

Kinsella, E. A. (2001). Reflections on reflective practice. *Canadian Journal of Occupational Therapy*, *68*(3), 195–198.

Lambert, H. (2006). Accounting for EBM: notions of evidence in medicine. *Social Science & Medicine*, *62*(11), 2633–2645.

Mattingly, C. (1991). The narrative nature of clinical reasoning. *American Journal of Occupational Therapy*, *45*(11), 998–1005.

Mattingly, C., & Fleming, M. H. (1994). *Clinical reasoning: Forms of inquiry in therapeutic practice.* F.A. Davis Company.

McIntosh, J., Marques, B., & Mwipiko, R. (2021). Therapeutic landscapes and indigenous culture: Māori health models in Aotearoa/New Zealand. In J. C. Spee, A. McMurray, & M. McMillan (Eds.), *Clan and tribal perspectives on social, economic and environmental sustainability: Indigenous stories from around the globe* (pp. 143–158). Emerald Publishing Limited.

Pandit, M. (2020). Critical factors for successful management of VUCA times. *BMJ Leader.* http://dx.doi.org/10.1136/leader-2020-000305

Rogers, C. R. (1951). *Client-centered therapy: Its current practice, implications, and theory.* Riverside Press.

Schön, D. (1983). *The reflective practitioner: How professionals think in action.* Basic Books.

Skinner, E. H., Haines, K. J., Hayes, K., Seller, D., Toohey, J. C., Reeve, J. C., Holdsworth, C., & Haines, T. P. (2015). Future of specialised roles in allied health practice: who is responsible? *Australian Health Review, 39*(3), 255–259.

Taylor, M. C. (2000). *Evidence-based practice for occupational therapists.* Wiley-Blackwell.

Thoma, A., & Eaves, F. F., III (2015). A brief history of evidence-based medicine (EBM) and the contributions of Dr David Sackett. *Aesthetic Surgery Journal, 35*(8), 261–263.

Wasserman, J. A., & Loftus, S. (2019). Changing demographic and cultural dimensions of populations: implications for health care and decision making. In J. Higgs, G. M. Jensen, S. Loftus, & N. Christensen (Eds.), *Clinical reasoning in health professions* (pp. 87–96). Elsevier.

Wieringa, S., & Greenhalgh, T. (2015). 10 years of mindlines: a systematic review and commentary. *Implementation Science, 10*, 45.

CHAPTER 2

The Five Finger Framework: Development and Rationale

Fostering Thinking Skills

Jan Hendrik Roodt[1] and Linda Robertson[2]

[1]Advanced Academic, Facilitator, Te Pūkenga, New Zealand
[2]Associate Professor Emeritus, Occupational Therapy, Te Pūkenga, New Zealand

INTRODUCTION

Client interactions, making decisions, and taking relevant action occupy the days of professionals in service enterprises such as occupational therapy, social work, and nursing. This also extends to teaching, engineering professions, and systems design. As we grow and progress in our professional fields, we become more accomplished at the daily tasks. However, where do novices start, and how do practitioners deal with the rapidly changing world that is increasingly volatile, uncertain, and ambiguous?

This chapter introduces the Five Finger Framework (FFF), building upon the historic concepts discussed within Chapter 1. We begin by examining the modern practice environment, followed by an exploration of evidence-based practice (EBP) and its complexities. The notion of artful and situated practice is introduced. It involves integrating critical reflective practice, continuous transformative learning, and anticipatory thinking. The motivations behind practicing mindfully, including the concept of moral empathy, are explored. Additionally, the factors that facilitate or hinder critical reflective practice are discussed.

Next, development of the FFF based on current research findings is covered. To provide context for the discussion, we briefly touch upon the relevant research and outcomes that were published, presented, and tested in New Zealand. Then the use of the hand and fingers as metaphor is explored within the pedagogical context.

The chapter concludes by providing a concise description of the hand, palm, and five finger metaphor and introducing how evidence can be utilized to support reasoning and action in EBP.

Professional Reasoning in Healthcare: Navigating Uncertainty Using the Five Finger Framework, First Edition.
Edited by Helen Jeffery, Linda Robertson, Jan Hendrik Roodt, and Susan Ryan.

THE COMPLEXITY OF PRACTICE DRIVES THE NEED FOR PROFESSIONAL REASONING SKILLS

Practitioners face a growing challenge due to the increasing complexity, volatility, and uncertainty in their work environments. The situation is largely driven by the rapid socio-technological changes observed in what is commonly referred to as the "Second Machine Age" (Brynjolfsson & McAfee, 2016). They must now navigate diverse stakeholder expectations, ranging from practice-specific considerations to broader concerns such as finance, environmental sustainability, regulatory compliance, employment matters, and political imperatives. This necessitates the development of heightened sense-making abilities and high-level thinking skills (Bannigan & Moores, 2009; Turner, 2019) to deliver quality outcomes for clients.

The quality of professional work depends on how practice is motivated, designed, and evaluated, all with a focus on achieving positive outcomes for the clients. In this context, quality refers to the extent to which interventions are comprehensive, justified, and beneficial for the clients. This understanding takes into consideration the specific circumstances and is documented and agreed upon by all relevant parties. It is also reflected in the execution of the intervention.

For instance, reasoning in practice can be seen as a technical rational process that relies on evidence. It involves following established routines and behaviors to provide services to clients. This approach aims to minimize risks and ensure accountability by adhering to established rules and protocols (Rolfe et al., 2010). The search for evidence to support professional practice is influenced by beliefs regarding what constitutes effective and valuable practice.

The technical rational approach involves applying a set of predetermined rules or procedures, derived from research, as a formula for practice. The assumption is that following established rules and protocols ensures efficient and effective service delivery. It relies on a belief that practice can be standardized and made predictable through adherence to these rules.

However, accomplished practitioners may also view practice as a rational artful endeavor, where professional judgment and intuition play essential roles. Here, the argument is that practice is characterized by a lack of predictability, requiring professionals to make complex decisions that rely on a combination of professional judgment, intuition, and common sense. According to this approach, professionals need to be adaptable and flexible in their knowledge application, identifying and utilizing principles as appropriate to each unique situation. In unexpected circumstances, rigid rules may not provide helpful guidance, and professionals must rely on "a mixture of professional judgment, intuition and common sense" (Fish & Coles, 1998, p. 32).

Views of Reasoning

In nursing literature, two views of reasoning have been described as "the external, scientific and the internal, intuitive" (Rycroft-Malone et al., 2009, p. 81). The external, scientific approach to care involves relying on evidence-based knowledge and established guidelines in practice. The focus is on the use of external sources, such as research findings and standardized protocols, to guide decision making and actions. It values the systematic application of scientific evidence to provide consistent and reliable care to patients. On the other hand, the internal, intuitive approach recognizes the importance of healthcare professionals' personal experiences, judgment, and intuition in practice. Practitioners employing this approach interpret external sources by engaging their tacit knowledge (knowing *why* rather than knowing *what* – a combination of experience, insight, and intuition) and understanding of the context and patient needs. Those individuals can make quick decisions and take appropriate actions based on a combination of intuition, reflection, and on-the-spot experimentation.

Schön (1983) originally introduced the concept of reflection-in-action, which emphasizes being mindful in the moment of action and considering not only what needs to be done but also why. The artful practitioner engages in reflection, on-the-spot experimentation, and action, using a model of "knowing in action" (Rolfe et al., 2010, p. 168). At this advanced level of practice, professionals may possess a deep understanding of their patients and situations and make intuitive decisions without consciously knowing the basis for their knowledge. They become situated and embodied in the sense-making and meaning-making processes of interventions.

While the discussion has primarily focused on healthcare practice, we recognize that professional reasoning is relevant to all fields and disciplines. In the field of system design engineering, the ability to adopt a broad perspective and handle unforeseen circumstances is a crucial aspect of professional artistry. Buede and Miller (2016, p. 5) argue that "big picture people" or holistic practitioners in engineering possess this skill set. These professionals are adept at considering multiple factors, understanding the interconnectedness of system components, and incorporating a comprehensive perspective into their work. As a result, at the graduate level of engineering education, critical thinking skills are increasingly emphasized. These skills go beyond technical knowledge and encompass aspects such as fairness, precision, and logic in the testing, identifying, and evaluation of assumptions, concepts, and information. Ralston and Bays (2013) highlight the integration of these intellectual traits into engineering training, aiming to cultivate qualities such as humility, integrity, intellectual empathy, and intellectual perseverance.

Thus, professional reasoning skills play a vital role in developing expertise and ensuring high-quality practice under uncertainty and in complex environments. The skills involve the ability to gather and critically evaluate information, make sound judgments, and consider the broader implications of one's decisions and actions. Honing these skills is indispensable for professionals to navigate complex and unpredictable situations, address challenges and achieve positive outcomes within their respective domains. Incorporating professional reasoning into education and training enables undergraduate students to acquire the necessary skills and perspectives to excel in their chosen professions.

EVIDENCE-BASED PRACTICE

The EBP movement has provided many challenges for professionals in relation to translating evidence into care. For instance, when general practitioners (GPs) felt that their traditional role was being challenged in the 1980s, a model of evidence-based medicine (EBM) was developed that was thought to reflect real-world practice more accurately. The three components were:

1. Mindfulness in one's approach toward EBM itself, and to the influences on decision making.
2. Pragmatism – in one's approach to finding and evaluating evidence; and

3. Knowledge of the patient – as the most useful resource in effective communication of evidence (Galbraith et al., 2017, p. 1).

Rycroft-Malone et al. (2009) outlined four types of evidence in nursing practice: research, clinical experience, patient experience, and information from the local context. Interestingly, these two summaries of being evidence based propose different perspectives: one is focused on the attitude of the professional toward sources of evidence while the second is focused on the sources themselves. These views are examples of how two different health professional groups have dealt with making sense of EBP in their practice.

Common concerns are the resistance toward the research taking center stage, and the inclusion of the patient as a key factor. The differences are the pragmatic concerns of nursing toward being contextually relevant as well as acknowledging the impact of the experience that the practitioner brings; the GP account reflects a more philosophical approach to the interaction between the clinician and their task to deliver practice that stems from an evidence orientation. These two examples are interesting accounts of how professional groups are grappling with the need to make sense of how they integrate evidence within their practice. These views, however, do reflect the widespread acceptance of the importance of being evidence based even though there are differences in the way this might be conceptualized. The greatest impact on professionals' intentions to engage in EBP behaviors has been reported to be the factors specific to healthcare organizations (Klaic et al., 2019).

The interplay between environmental factors and personal skills in successful EBP implementation has been highlighted by Whiteside et al. (2016), who note that despite potential challenges within the organizational environment, experienced practitioners can still effectively integrate EBP into their routine practice. This suggests that both organizational support and the professional's critical analysis skills and intentions are essential factors in the adoption and sustainability of EBP. We consider these two aspects in more detail below.

Organizational Support

Van Woerkom and Croon (2008) pointed out that limited work had been done on critical reflection in the context of the formal workplace and initiated understanding of reflective working. They drew on Schön's (1983) work to explore how reflection-on-work and reflection-in-work may be used to improve performance and the quality of a service and suggest that the essential components include the following.

- Willingness to be open about mistakes in the context of sharing with peers.
- Asking for feedback as part of learning.
- Trying new ways of working: experimentation – hypothesis setting and testing as part of reflection-in-work.
- Criticality in answering the "why" related to justification for the premises of posed problems and possible solutions, including sociopolitical questioning of the status quo and those elements taken for granted.
- Challenging group think.
- Awareness of one's identity as a practitioner, asking questions about who one wants to be as a professional and understanding one's motives for being part of the profession.

Interestingly, many employees in the study felt that they fell far short of critical reflective workplace practice as a result of low job autonomy and lack of opportunity for taking initiative.

Individual Professional Skills

In relation to how the intention of the practitioner affects the evidence brought to reviewing practice, Gambrill (2018, p. 113), in her work related to the reasoning skills of social workers, identifies two key points.

- One is that an essential aspect of EBP is the health professional who brings "values, knowledge, and skills integral to the process of EBP . . . including recognizing ignorance."
- Her second main point, supported by Van Woerkom and Croon (2008), emphasizes the necessity of developing cultures of inquiry. Within these cultures, participants are encouraged to engage in active open-minded thinking to critically appraise claims, gather and collate important questions that emerge, involve clients as informed participants, and enhance transparency regarding the actions taken and their resulting effects.

Clearly, EBP is an active process that entails both searching for established knowledge and exploring areas that remain unknown. While relevant research can provide solutions to uncertainties, there are instances where a lack of research necessitates the use of well-argued theories and practical experiences to justify practice. Sniderman et al. (2013) highlight that due to limitations in available research evidence, "clinicians must still reason through the best choices for an individual because even in the absence of full and secure knowledge, clinical decisions must still be made" (p. 1108).

Supporting the notion of practitioners needing to develop critical reasoning skills, the concept of "mindlines" suggests that the number of guidelines on any given topic will continue to expand because new individual realities and scientific paradigms constantly emerge (Gabbay & le May, 2004; Wieringa & Greenhalgh, 2015). From the early promotion of EBP, it has been recognized that critical reasoning skills are necessary to integrate clinical expertise with the best external evidence (Sackett et al., 1996). EBP extends beyond utilizing literature as evidence and requires the ability to navigate and incorporate various forms of evidence into decision-making processes. It is suggested that in medicine, there is a mixture of skills and uncertainties that are grounded in medical knowledge but could be more accurately called "evidence-based clinical judgment" (Timmermans & Angell, 2001, p. 354).

The Role of Tacit Knowledge in Evidence-based Practice

The interplay between procedural reasoning and tacit knowledge is of concern. Tacit knowledge, which develops over time through personal experience, plays a significant role in decision-making processes and can override protocols and guidelines. It helps practitioners align the underlying protocols and procedures of practice with the specific beliefs and circumstances of individuals. Flynn et al. (2012) provide examples of this phenomenon in their study of the Barthel index as an outcome measure. Clinicians adjusted the scores based on their "clinical judgment and contextual circumstances" (p. 77), demonstrating the impact of tacit knowledge on the standards.

The understanding brought by clients is another crucial aspect influenced by tacit knowledge. In a study on cancer patients' views of effective interventions, the measure of treatment success was often expressed as "feeling better in myself" (Broom & Tovey, 2012, p. 149). This was influenced by previous experiences with medical interventions, indicating that clients' decisions "are mediated by a range of personal and social processes" (p. 152). The client's cultural perspectives also play a significant role in shaping understanding and cooperation with desired treatment plans. For example, excluding the family from decisions regarding intervention and discharge can lead to anger and resistance, as it may be perceived as disrespectful to the family, even if the client has apparent decision-making autonomy.

Similarly, cultural perspectives shape practitioners' perceptions of individuals and impact clients' attitudes toward medical care and their ability to understand, manage, and cope with illness (Mankar & Shaik, 2021). Awareness of the influence of cultural perspectives on healthcare is crucial to ensure effective and respectful practice. Specific practice models have been developed to guide clinical assessments and interventions within particular cultural contexts. An example is the Meihena model designed when working with Māori, the Indigenous people of New Zealand, which recognizes and respects the cultural values and beliefs of this specific population (Pitama et al., 2017). Such models provide a framework for healthcare professionals to understand and address the unique needs and preferences of diverse cultural groups, fostering culturally responsive care and, importantly, enabling Indigenous practitioners to practice in a way that is a good fit with their own culture.

In conclusion, we note that while there is general agreement that EBP is more than utilizing research evidence, there is limited clarity regarding what constitutes "other" evidence, and insufficient attention given to how such evidence is gathered and integrated into decision making and student learning. The broader concept of evidence encompasses not only research findings but also well-supported theories, client satisfaction, and practitioners' experiential knowledge. Exploring current perspectives on critical thinking and strategies for gathering evidence and developing experiential knowledge will be discussed as we introduce the FFF as an instrument for considering and gathering evidence toward decision-making and action.

THE FIVE FINGER FRAMEWORK

Context and Motivation

Novice practitioners, including students and new graduates, lack extensive experience in their respective fields, so they are limited in using practice knowledge to support their reasoning. However, they do have the potential to develop critical thinking skills and make informed decisions based on the available evidence. These practitioners can learn to make better sense of the situations they face. They can develop the skills to analyze and evaluate the available evidence effectively, and while formal research critique is an important aspect of their education, it is equally crucial that they understand how to recognize and develop sound arguments for practice decisions.

Promoting a reflective approach is a key aspect of professional development. It is essential to understand what motivates therapists to engage in critical reflection. Robertson et al. (2013) highlight the importance of addressing this fundamental question. By exploring the underlying motivations, educators and practitioners can better support therapists in developing a critically reflective mindset. Understanding the driving forces behind reflective practice can lead to enhanced engagement and application of critical thinking skills that will stand practitioners in good stead throughout their career. Driving forces include curiosity, a thirst to analyze how knowledge is constructed and habitually using past and present knowledge to develop new mental models that provide a variety of understandings of practice.

Three broad motivators for the development of artful practice that have affected the development of the FFF have been postulated.

1. Critical reflectivity as a crucial part of transformative learning.
2. Transformative learning and development of strong models of practice.
3. Sense-making and anticipatory thinking.

We now briefly discuss these three concepts before we introduce the research for the development of the FFF.

Critical Reflectivity

Being able to think critically allows one to solve problems in an equitable and effective manner. Critical thinking consists of specific skills enabling one to:

- analyze information,
- make inferences,
- judge and evaluate concepts,
- make decisions, and
- solve problems and address complex issues.

Besides cognitive skills like retrieving information from memory in a selective manner and visualizing concepts, critical thinking includes a certain attitude,

according to Snyder and Snyder (2008). Such an attitude consists of the need to be well informed, to have an inquisitive mind, a drive for being fair, and an openness to diverse viewpoints. Rodgers (2002) considered definitions and descriptions of reflective thinking. Four main points emerged, including:

- valuing of intellectual growth for all,
- using systematic and disciplined ways of thinking,
- seeing reflection as part of sense making and meaning making,
- being situated in conversation with the self and others.

Engaging in critical reflection is not a simple or effortless process, as highlighted by Mälkki (2010). According to Mezirow (2018), critical reflectivity plays a crucial role in transformative learning, requiring an emotional connection and deep structural shifts in our thoughts and feelings. This suggests that critically assessing our beliefs and perspectives and shifting our reality are often motivated by the necessity for change and the management of risks and uncertainties. And in everyday practice, practitioners may fall victim to cognitive biases and external pressures from the working environment and the routine cases they encounter. For instance, the pressure to discharge clients rapidly can dominate practice and lead to shortcuts and an approach where the pressure for early discharge overrides client and health professional concerns re timely discharge. A study conducted in Australia in 2019 also revealed a perceived incongruence between clinical reasoning and reflective practice among participants. In everyday practice, therapists often have limited opportunities to articulate their values and beliefs as part of their reasoning process (Knightbridge, 2019). Nevertheless, participants in the same study acknowledged that reflective practice enhances the safety and quality of service delivery.

Taylor (2014) proposes a more enduring motivation for critical reflection, building on Mälkki's work. Taylor argued that a dynamic and congruent relationship exists between critical reflection and empathy. Empathy enables individuals to adopt the perspective of others, leading to a deeper understanding. It involves an interdependence between cognition and unconscious emotional responses. This connection between emotions, moral and ethical foundations (moral empathy), and the ability to critically reflect and make sense at the cognitive level supports therapists' motivation to better understand their clients. While moral empathy is an innate capacity that varies among individuals (Pieris et al., 2022), it can be nurtured through reflective practice, enabling practitioners to form meaningful connections with patients and enhance their overall professional growth.

Although it can be argued that the motivation for engaging in critical thinking and reflective practice stems from moral and ethical considerations, there are two main schools of thought regarding critical thinking skills. Monteiro et al. (2020) emphasize the significance of expertise that is developed through practice, built upon both formalized and experiential knowledge. They argue that possessing a vast, well-organized, and accessible body of knowledge specific to the field is essential for effective practice. However, other scholars view critical thinking as a set of general and transferable skills, such as judgmental framing, analysis, evaluation, and synthesis (Abrami et al., 2008). They believe that formalized knowledge in the field has equal importance alongside these critical thinking skills. So, perspectives differ between the significance of deep knowledge specific to the field and the general and transferable skills associated with critical thinking. Both perspectives contribute valuable insights into transformative learning and the development of expertise and effective practice.

Transformative Learning

Supporting professional development and continuous education in a fast-paced world involves recognizing the dynamic nature of knowledge and emphasizing the integration of field-specific knowledge and practice (Lester, 1995). This experiential learning must ensure that professionals are equipped with the skills and up-to-date knowledge to thrive in a changing environment. It is an ongoing process and according to Dewey (1981, p. 450), "education must be conceived as a continuing reconstruction of experience." Dewey based this statement on the belief that ongoing learning is concerned with developing new attitudes to novel experiences. Reflective thought and practice, as defined by Dewey (1910), involve challenging existing worldviews and beliefs, generating knowledge within a social and cultural context, and enhancing critical thinking skills.

Mezirow (2018) described this process of transforming mindsets, meanings, assumptions, and expectations as transformative learning. Transformative learning is a key objective of reflective practice because it "helps us critique our own thought processes, our points of view and the fields that shaped them" (Christie et al., 2015, p. 22). It fosters the ability to gain perspective, make informed decisions, and improve interventions. Bransford and Schwartz (1999) emphasize the importance of extensive contextual knowledge in both reflective practice and critical thinking. Mezirow (2018) cautions that an exclusive focus on contextual issues should be avoided. Furthermore, in Blair and Robertson's (2005) exploration of challenges for curriculum planners in health and social care courses, they noted that a major challenge is to ensure that "students have the opportunity to analyze how knowledge is constructed and where power resides" (p. 275). Their observation is that there is a definite preference for literature on EBP when compared to that arising from reflective or reflexive practice, thus indicating that social reality has not been well captured in the curriculum. To aid in the integration of disciplinary knowledge, professional practice context and reflexive processes, Harrison (2021) proposed a learning approach that makes learners and practitioners aware of the different aspects of their practice and how their experiential knowledge develops. His capability development model focuses on pointing out the iterative interaction between field-specific knowledge and more general reflective processes.

Turning now to the process of interaction with the field of practice, our discussion moves to sense making and anticipatory thinking and action.

Sense Making and Anticipatory Thinking

We all need to make sense of the world in which we live and to act in ways that enforce our ability to deal with challenges (Rodgers, 2008). The challenges may be of a personal and of a professional nature. For example, we may face a client situation that is very different from what we have experienced before, or we may be surprised by a situation that evolves and becomes very different from our expectations. This sense-making process is rather complex and can be explained in part from Dewey's perspective of ongoing reconstruction of experiences.

Sense making is a mental process that considers past experiences and current knowledge and reinterprets this

to rationalize current situations and the actions of people (Weick et al., 2005). It explains events and trouble-shoots problems. The sense-making process constantly constructs a model of individual experience that becomes a practice worldview – a mental model. This mental model is forever changing in a recursive manner. All elements of the process are interdependent, call on each other and themselves for development, and emerge simultaneously (Morin, 2008).

Although sense making can take the form of explaining events and situations, one can also develop sense about future situations. We learn to anticipate future challenges and identify opportunities. Klein et al. (2010) call this anticipatory thinking. They point out that it is a form of problem and opportunity detection that is essential to planning and critical to coordination of activities. Weak or underdeveloped mental models limit all forms of sense making and negatively impact practice.

In conclusion, to appreciate the complexity of practice and to develop richer mental models, all practitioners can benefit from developing all aspects of critical reflective practice. We now present an overview of the FFF and its contribution to critical reflective practice. The research that led to the development of the FFF is discussed next, followed by pedagogical considerations of the use of metaphor and, finally, justification for the use of the FFF.

Research Toward Development of the Five Finger Framework

Professionals use a broad scope of knowledge in their construction of EBP. Reasoning about action requires skills in identifying appropriate sources of information and judging their impact on the situation. It takes account of an extensive array of factors such as the client's circumstances, their needs and opinions, the professional's knowledge, the workplace culture, and the available resources. This diverse knowledge base must be understood and be familiar to students and novice practitioners if it is to be used effectively. Broom and Adams (2012) note that "clinicians are faced with the plethora of ideological, epistemological and practical issues" where value judgments are required to manage such aspects as the "quality of evidence, risks, costs, and patient preference" (p. 9).

To identify the essential skills and strategies currently used in practice, a research project was undertaken. Two issues directed the research.

- The first was to better understand the evidence that was suitable for practice in the current environment.
- The second was the rather confronting evidence that new graduates are reluctant to even consider looking for evidence unless guided by a supervisor and that they lose these skills quickly after becoming qualified (Klaic et al., 2018).

Qualitative data was gathered through interviews and focus groups involving practitioners, final year students, and new graduates. The study identified that there was a great diversity of thinking about the essentials of EBP varying on a continuum from finding and applying the outcomes literature to being prepared to change thinking on the basis of what works.

Although critiquing research is the most studied aspect of learning how to be evidence based, therapists did not spend a lot of time looking for and critiquing research which is consistent with many studies of EBP (for an example see Benfield & Jeffery, 2022). One approach was to use their own practice experiences and to seek feedback on case management from colleagues. Essential features of being evidence based included asking relevant questions, being open to challenge, and receiving and using feedback. These elements were identified as being an area of weakness in the students (Jeffery et al., 2020).

The results of the study were a stimulus for the development of five key topics for encapsulation in the FFF. The practitioner is included as an integral component of the framework and acknowledges the influence that the knowledge and skills of the professional have on the effective integration of the other four components in the framework. The five components are discussed in detail within subsequent chapters. Besides the use of personal knowledge and experience, the practitioner considers (touches base with) four other sources of information (see Figure 2.1): the expertise of others, client insights, policy and local context, and curated knowledge including literature. The transformation of knowledge and arguments about action are recursive processes that are part of sense making (explaining and diagnosing) and anticipatory thinking (formulating expectations and possible outcomes).

The framework was introduced in the Te Pūkenga occupational therapy school (New Zealand) and with postgraduate students from a range of disciplines. Results were presented at conferences to a range of allied health professionals. Feedback from professional educators, practitioners, and students was that the simplicity of the framework provided an appealing visual overview of the elements needing to be considered in a comprehensive view of evidence.

The Pedagogical Metaphor – The Active Hand and Fingers

Active embodiment and engagement in practical work, along with the pragmatic application of knowledge, are crucial because the

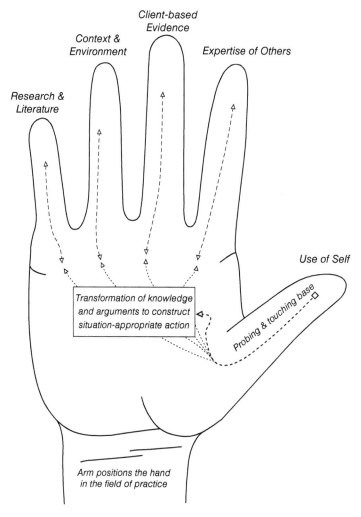

Research &
Literature

Context &
Environment

Client-based
Evidence

Expertise of Others

Use of Self

Transformation of knowledge
and arguments to construct
situation-appropriate action

Probing & touching base

Arm positions the hand
in the field of practice

FIGURE 2.1   The Five Finger Framework and the metaphor of the hand.

effective application of knowledge serves as the measure of its worth. The goal with the FFF is to provide support to graduate students and clinical practitioners, enabling them to cultivate their practice and expand their knowledge in a structured manner. To this end, metaphors play a vital role in comprehending and explaining intricate ideas (Snowden, 2000).

Many educational theories rely on metaphors and emphasize taking action (Botha, 2009). Metaphors not only establish and represent values and perspectives but also convey epistemic content. They facilitate the transfer of meaning from something familiar to something unknown or abstract, allowing for visualization of complex concepts. To enable this transition and unlock the potential for transformative practice, effective metaphors incorporate visually evocative and symbolic elements that connect to the fundamental aspects of the values, practice, and knowledge in a particular field. In this instance, the active practitioner hand was introduced as a familiar concept representing the elements of thought and practice that are essential to evidence-based professional reasoning.

In the FFF, the five fingers represent five areas to remember to think about, starting with who the practitioner is, what they know, and how they operate (the thumb in Figure 2.1). This simple comparison draws a parallel between the hand, composed of four fingers and a thumb, and EBP which, based on our research, consists of five essential components that must coexist for optimal functionality.

The hand as a metaphor reflects the complexity of the compound movements and the incredible dexterity needed for the hand to be an effective precision tool. Each finger contributes to the strength of the hand in different proportions and the thumb interacts with (touches) the fingers to ensure a grip that meets the functional requirements. A complex array of muscles, tendons, and nerves must be coordinated to ensure the grip is effective. Likewise, the reasoning of the health professional integrates sources of information that contribute to the requirements of decision making. All sources ("fingers") must engage repeatedly with the thumb to make effective decisions. How well the practitioner interprets each new scenario is dependent on the "world within," i.e., previous experience determines the way new situations are manipulated (the thumb). This is like having a memory of movement and sensation which enables overall function. If the thumb continues to touch base with the fingers, then the overall strength of the hand is maintained (and professional competence continues to develop). If one or more of the fingers are routinely missed, then the hand becomes unbalanced and atrophies. The five fingers are about "grasping" ideas and information and bringing them together in the palm to create well-informed decision making while transforming knowledge. Each person has a hand that has unique features so decision-making processes may differ depending on what informs them. What is important is that reasoning is well informed and routinely used, becoming a habit to both explain and anticipate situations.

Justification for Use of the Five Finger Framework

Reviews of EBP indicate that an inclusive framework is needed to capture the realities of how outcomes are achieved. A well-researched example of this is the PARIHS framework (Promoting Action on Research Implementation in Health Services) which has been developed for health professionals. In this, evidence is knowledge that has been located from a variety of sources, tested and found to be credible. More specifically, the PARIHS framework identifies these sources as research, clinical experience, patient experience, and local data/information. However, a framework that is comprehensive, with extensive research to justify its value, has its problems. This framework has been found to be very cumbersome, resulting in shortcuts being taken and the value of the framework lost in the difficulty of applying it (Rycroft-Malone, 2004).

While PARIHS does consider the broad context of the interventions, it recognizes that implementation of research evidence is problematic because of the dynamic and complex practice environment (Rycroft-Malone, 2004). Conceivably using a quantitative, focused approach is never going to capture this complexity. Consequently, professionals need to have an alternative approach to pay attention to all elements of evidence, make sense of it, and communicate it effectively to stakeholders. This is consistent with Wieringa and Greenhalgh's (2015) stance that the concept of mindlines should be developed further to "produce richer sources of evidence-based knowledge" (p. 1).

In the FFF, complexity is captured in the broad directives provided by the five fingers. In one sense, it includes greater complexity when compared to the PARIHS: the professional is included as being influential in the evidence-based approach as they will determine the information used to underpin the best outcomes for the scenario being considered. Moreover, it has the four components that are generally identified in the research: literature, the client, the context, and the views of experienced professionals. An example of these components of evidence in occupational therapy is provided by Hoffman et al. (2017) who state that: "Evidence-based occupational therapists use clinical reasoning to integrate information from four sources: their clinical experience, research evidence, client values and circumstances, and the practice context" (p. 4).

In their work on applying self-determination theory to professional reasoning in occupational therapy, Bolton and Dean (2018) refer to the importance of experiential learning to develop reasoning skills. However, they indicate that there is a "lack of a framework" (p. 3) for enhancing instructional strategies in teaching. The FFF is such a framework. It has the potential to direct students' thoughts to specific components of practice, providing a way of thinking that will affect both their planning for practice and their reflections on practice. This strategy could readily enhance the depth of reflection on practice that is central to a self-determination approach. They would be seeing themselves as the "thumb" of the FFF, i.e., the practitioner/student who makes sense of the other four fingers to work out what to do in the first instance and then to consider how well it was done and what was learned. The FFF spells out what is integral to practice knowledge and it enables the user to modify the questions related to each finger, thus providing a focus for a particular learning exercise or personal reflection.

Reasoning and Taking Action

A professional reasoning structure and EBP are connected through the focus on interventions toward a quality outcome for a client. The critical thinking and collection of relevant information lead to practical and considered action. They take place within an ethical framework of responsibility and provisionality. Provisionality involves recognizing that a solution is linked to a specific time, available knowledge, and situation. Any solution remains open to change in the future (Andersson & Törnberg, 2018; Woermann & Cilliers, 2012).

Unsworth (2018) also considers the nexus between reasoning, decision making, and practice: "Clinicians must be judicious in selecting and using the best evidence" (p. 479). The FFF supports the practitioner to do just that. Using reasoning frameworks in conjunction with the FFF, a set of congruent arguments to support the client can be developed. Recognizing that reasoning under complexity has its limits, the value of structured approaches is discussed next and is concluded with a simple summary of the FFF in terms of a generic reasoning schema.

Toward Reflective Practice and Sharing of Experience

Skilled practitioners with experiential knowledge often consider their own experience, historical cases, and other sources to initiate the process of devising interventions. The novice practitioner has limited experience and must rely on directed and structured learning approaches to grow their skills. For experience and formal learning to be shaped into experiential knowledge, sense making and meaning making must take place. This process is based on an experience in a field, reflection on the experience, and making links to other experiences (Tonelli & Shapiro, 2020). When faced with a new practice situation, the practitioner speculates about a plausible explanation of what is presented and considers reasonable actions toward a positive outcome. This may include asking for support from peers, looking at recorded notes, and engaging with the client.

By using frameworks like the FFF, it is possible to gather and consider a broad range of information in a structured manner. The practitioner, when faced with a new client, may have a hunch of how to address the issue and solve the problem. The processes of sense making and critical thinking come into play and a claim develops, based on experiential knowledge. A plausible intervention is considered in terms of actions, monitoring, and judging of the likely outcomes. The practitioner may find it useful to discuss aspects of the case with a peer or supervisor before and after meeting with the client. With the insights gained from the client interaction, regulatory and other concerns may be raised. In some instances, literature on similar cases may also provide insight. Part of the structuring of information, at any point in the act of practice and critical reflection, is to consider how the information pieces fit together to support a logical path of action toward an anticipated quality outcome.

Toulmin recognized the need for a simple structure to organize information to validate claims (Karbach, 1987; Voss et al., 1993). The essence of the structure is similar to the thought processes discussed above.

- It starts by considering a claim in the form of an assertion (*the client needs a hoist for lifting onto a bed*).
- Grounds are furnished for the claim (*the client cannot get onto the bed by themselves, the family is unable to assist physically, hoists have been used successfully in similar situations*).

- A qualifier modifies the scope of the claim (*in the short term, as hoists are expensive and are often rented for a short time*).
- A rebuttal is introduced to acknowledge exceptions or information that may invalidate the claim (*unless the client lives upstairs and a hoist is too heavy according to local building codes*).

Using the FFF, the practitioner can also keep a reflective journal for sharing with others and as evidence of the process followed to construct an intervention. The use of a reflective framework was shown in several studies to improve meaning making from challenging experiences (Markkanen et al., 2020).

Endsley (2001) states that experience and expertise play a major role in situation awareness, which can be defined as "the perception of the elements in the environment within a volume of time and space, the comprehension of their meaning and the projection of their status in the near future" (p. 4). Practical experience supports the development of long-term memory structures, which aid in recognizing patterns in the environment and have the effect of minimizing short-term working memory effort. As the practitioner's experiential knowledge grows, constructing evidence-based interventions and reflection may become more fluent. Skilled professionals recognize patterns faster, become confident of discerning nuanced differences between cases, and develop judgment of patient progress (Tonelli & Shapiro, 2020).

Recognizing Limits to Reasoning on Complex Issues and Automation

Over the years, several attempts have been made to augment practice by including automated reasoning engines to deal with the complexity and speed up delivery.

Examples of such reasoning engines include the use of advanced statistical processing programs, deep-learning computational artificial intelligence, and computer simulations in providing diverse clinical information and decision support. Incorporating these tools into everyday workflows remains challenging (Elstein et al., 1990; Li et al., 2022; Liaw et al., 2022; Rodrigues et al., 2022; Zhang & Li, 2022). There are several arguments to consider when contemplating the use of these technologies to augment human practice.

Development of a strong level of skilled practice, and even more so artful practice, is known to be a slow and deliberate process of experiential learning. But time spent by a human practitioner on practical tasks is crucial and artful practice is achieved through a host of mechanisms. This includes client interaction, peer review, case study, publication review, and professional responsibility (Abrandt Dahlgren et al., 2022; Elstein et al., 1990). The practitioner is often required to consider alternatives and, on the face of it, evaluate and judge equally valid solutions (Schraw et al., 1995).

Practitioners also see consultation with a client as a complex process happening within a limited timeframe. Within this setting, they must "discover solutions to health and social problems" as they gain trust from the client and consider the client perspectives on their own needs and path to recovery (Innes, 2007, p. 61). It takes time to develop a likely explanation of the situation and to propose an initial intervention (Thompson, 2012). The process is highly nonlinear. Atkinson and Nixon-Cave (2011) state that iterative cycles of development take place based on:

- observation and impressions,
- information gathering,
- diagnosis and treatment planning, and
- monitoring.

Spring et al. (2019) describe a similar overarching process of EBP that starts with asking a set of questions. The questions consider the patient-specific information and a plausible intervention that is front of mind. An intervention is considered and applied, evaluated, monitored, and adjusted as required. The complexity of the process is driven by uncertainty and ambiguity, part of the professional practice scenario, and this makes diagnosis, treatment, and plausible outcomes difficult to establish (Tonelli & Upshur, 2019). They assert "that the majority of the uncertainty faced by clinicians on a day-to-day basis is epistemic" (p. 508) and related to making sense of a variety of information sources.

With the advances reported since 2023 in language and narrative processing computational intelligence, we anticipate a resurgence of possible supporting technologies. Our position is that artful and situated practice includes aspects of judgment that will remain within the ambit of the professional human.

Exploring the Use of the Five Finger Framework

To explore the use of the FFF, one may start by considering the hand that is positioned by the arm to act in a field of practice like occupational therapy, design systems engineering, nursing, and so on. The profession provides the practitioner with a contextual position. Every hand has similar parts, but with unique features it has a practice identity.

The palm is bounded by the arches of the hand. The longitudinal arches down the fingers and the transverse arches across the metacarpal and carpal bones facilitate the function of the hand. In the FFF, the palm is a metaphor for the problem and resolution space which is created to facilitate reasoning, as discussed by Kassirer et al. (2010). Within this space, all the information from each of the five finger strands is brought together in an iterative manner. This allows for the relationship between them to be considered.

The degree, depth, and complexity of the reasoning remain with the reasoner and are dependent on their knowledge, ideas, and beliefs (Kassirer et al., 2010). Interpretations of a particular situation are likely to vary. The FFF encourages the reasoner to consider information drawn from five sources and look at the relationship between them. It promotes hypotheses generation and testing, thus developing a lateral approach to reasoning.

Broadley speaking, there are two types of problems. Some may be ill defined: they do not have clear goals or expected solutions. Others may be well defined with clear goals and well-defined outcomes. In her study on clinical reasoning, Mattingly (1994) notes that there is often a constant revision required as the therapist and client work together. This illustrates that the frequency of problems tends toward being ill defined. It has been shown that well-defined and ill-defined problems require separate cognitive processes and that epistemic beliefs play an important role in solving ill-defined problems (Schraw et al., 1995).

The initial construction of the problem and solution space is considered when the hand is placed into the practice domain and the *To What*, *With What*, and *For What* questions are raised to start the sense-making process (Weick, 2012). The practitioner starts with the cocreation and enacting (establishing) of the contextual environment by probing from experiential knowledge (Table 2.1). Situation awareness develops by considering the immediate data at their disposal, followed by evaluation of the developing information. A mental model of the situation takes shape (Endsley, 2001).

This is followed in Table 2.2 by considering the contribution of the fingers coming into play. Finally, in Table 2.3 the solution takes shape in the palm of the hand. The hand is transformed by the practice.

Starting with the practitioner "self," the initial situation is evaluated through a critical process of sense making and anticipating that a certain situation will unfold. Now, using the metaphor, the thumb assists the practitioner to manipulate, grasp, and refine decisions by obtaining relevant information from each of the fingers (Table 2.2). The skill of the practitioner is to be observant and ask the right questions.

The process of moving between the different fingers and the palm continues throughout the development and application of the intervention. The process is balanced by available resources and the questions of ethics, fairness, sustainability, and provisionality (Table 2.3). The character, the identity, of the practicing hand is changed through the process.

CONCLUDING REMARKS

This chapter has a strong focus on the complex environment, critical thinking skills, and awareness of how learning and construction of knowledge are supportive of sense making and anticipatory thinking. The debates around EBP continue. On the one hand, there is an argument that too much focus is placed on formalized knowledge, often overlooking the value of and need for experiential knowledge. On the other, experiential knowledge is seen as an outcome of the practice of deep knowledge in the field and that this knowledge always preceded the practical application. The position taken in this chapter is pragmatic: the careful and deliberate applications of know-how and know-why based on experience are equally important to a solid and current knowledge of the field of practice.

TABLE 2.1   The Hand is Positioned in the Field of Practice and the Problem Space

The Hand	The Hand is Positioned

Cocreating the environment
Situation awareness

Research & Literature

Context & Environment

Client-based Evidence

Expertise of Others

Use of Self

Transformation of knowledge and arguments to construct situation-appropriate action

Probing & touching base

Arm positions the hand in the field of practice

The hand is positioned into the context of the field of practice. The practitioner develops situation awareness by perceiving the elements presented about the client.

The questions to ask:
What is going on here?
What do I do next?

Think about this problem-structuring statement:
How do I attend TO the situation of the client, WITH the information at my disposal, FOR the purpose of action toward the broad GOAL of the client and my profession?

TABLE 2.2   The Five Fingers Come into Play

The Five Fingers	The Fingers in Action
Gathering, validating, and verifying information The judicious selection and use of best evidence	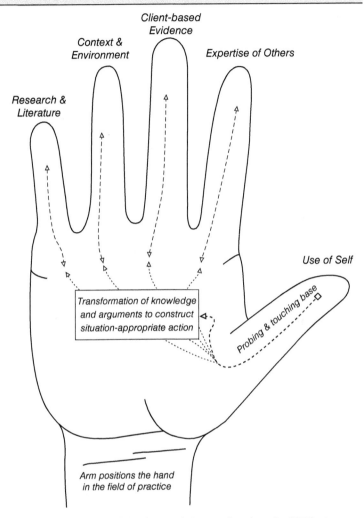

| **Thumb**
 Use of self | This is about you. What do you bring to the situation? What experience and knowledge inform your clinical reasoning? What attitudes and expectations do you have? The thumb assists the practitioner to grasp and refine decisions by obtaining relevant information from each of the fingers and synthesizing that information to create action that is a good fit with the situation and themselves. The skill of the practitioner is to ask the right questions.

 Questions to ask: *What is the hunch I have about this situation? What is familiar about this, what do I already know, what do I need to know and how can I find it out? What is my professional style and how can I make best use of myself in this situation?* |

(Continued)

TABLE 2.2 (Continued)

The Five Fingers	The Fingers in Action
Index finger Expertise of others	Expertise is developed through research and experience – the "know-how" that experienced practitioners hold is useful for the practitioner as is information from known experts in the field. Accessing knowledge from field experts can occur through online resources, presentations, and conferences, on-the-ground sharing of experiences, and judicious use of supervision. Using advise from experienced others in the workplace provides grounded ideas for specific practice situations and an immediate response. This finger provides certainty that reasoning is in keeping with current expectations and practice and can point to new directions. **Questions to ask:** *Who can help me with the decision, and how best can I access their expertise?*
Middle finger Client	The client (who may be individuals, groups, or communities) brings to the process essential understandings of what the problem is and what might work for them. Collaboration between client and practitioner profoundly influences the decisions made. **Questions to ask:** *What is the client perspective and situation? How can I best ascertain this and collaborate with them to good effect?*
Fourth finger Context and environment	Environment in this framework refers to both the practice environment and the community in which the setting is situated. The practitioner considers national and workplace protocols and procedures, cultural elements of the workplace and community, the resources available, and enablers and barriers to accessing those resources. **Questions to ask:** *How do I do things here, in this cultural context, in this place, and what can help me ascertain this?*
Little finger Research evidence, published literature, and curated wisdom	The research evidence refers to the underpinning theories that inform the profession and to current and emerging research that supports evolution of practice. The literature includes research articles, books, and reports that provide information about the value of an intervention. Critical appraisal is needed. What theories and models support practice? Curated cultural and Indigenous models of practice and generational wisdom may also contribute to the body of knowledge to be considered. **Questions to ask:** *What proven, reviewed, and validated knowledge can illuminate the issue I am facing? How can it inform my decision making and proposed intervention? How can the research and literature help me work out what to do and how to do it?*

TABLE 2.3   A Solution is Iteratively Crafted in the Palm of the Hand

The Hand and Palm	The Solution in the Palm

The palm
Transforming information and knowledge to deliver a solution

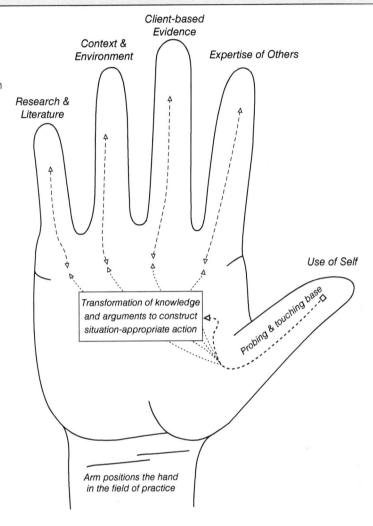

From the information gathered by the fingers, the situation-appropriate action/intervention is developed. As the intervention develops, it is prudent to include consideration of constraints and limitations.

Questions to ask in an iterative fashion:

Considering each finger, what evidence did I find to both inform and support my proposed intervention?

What evidence did I consider that hinted at a different solution and why did I discard that option?

If I ask "What could limit my solution – in terms of scope and time, for example?" of each finger, what qualifiers do I collect for my intervention?

If I ask "What may cause the intervention to be unsuitable in this situation?" by touching base with each finger, what may I discover that will render my solution invalid?

(Continued)

TABLE 2.3   (Continued)

The Hand and Palm	The Solution in the Palm
	If I finally ask "What future situation can I discover that may render my solution less than optimal?" what would each of the fingers tell me? What can I anticipate as future push-backs to my proposed solution? Am I relying on a solution that worked in the past while there may be a more suitable new option? Finally: Did I ask sufficient questions about the situation, the research, and my own skills and knowledge? What were my plans? What did I do and what outcomes were achieved? What was pivotal? What was redundant? What did I miss? What did I learn?
The hand My practice identity	**The questions to ask:** Am I practicing in an ethical manner and within the expectations of my profession? Am I operating in a fair and sustainable manner (working efficiently with resources, for example)? Have I considered the provisionality of my proposed actions? Can I say that I have pushed the boundaries to come up with a considered approach? Have I answered all the questions that I said would be important when developing the (clinical) question or description of the problem situation?

Still, the client must be the focus of attention and the reality is that there is a mix of students and novice practitioners, as well as skilled and artful professionals doing just that. The FFF is a response to the need for a simple and intuitive framework for dealing with growing knowledge loads and responsibilities where uncertainty and ambiguity rule. By showing how the FFF can be used to address the need for critical reflective practice, transformative learning, and sense making, the door is opened to a structured response to client needs (Figure 2.2). Through considering the hand metaphor, one can see how the FFF may be useful in a number of fields of practice. The aim remains to support judicious selection of evidence toward interventions that are fit for purpose for the client and within the regulatory and other constraints imposed on practice.

In the chapters that follow, each of the five information sources, or fingers, of the FFF is discussed in more detail. Narratives are used to draw on the power of story telling in facilitating learning. Narrative or story telling is helpful in that stories draw people in and provide an experience that is multisensorial and does not rely solely on cognition. The reader is able to relate to the story and assimilate the messages with their own situation and past experiences. Through narratives, the material is brought to life and the reader is shifted into the role of "actor" as they make links between the story and themselves (Clarke & Rossiter, 2008). The stories in this book help to bring theory to life, initiate the motivation to read, and illustrate the nuanced and complex elements that come together in the messiness of everyday professional reasoning.

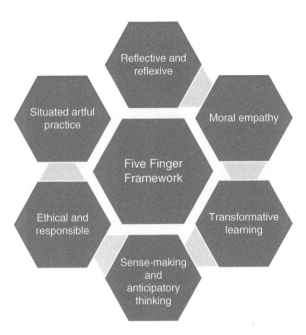

FIGURE 2.2   The Five Finger Framework overview.

REFERENCES

Abrami, P. C., Bernard, R. M., Borokhovski, E., Wade, A., Surkes, M. A., Tamim, R., & Zhang, D. (2008). Instructional interventions affecting critical thinking skills and dispositions: a stage 1 meta-analysis. *Review of Educational Research, 78*(4), 1102–1134.

Abrandt Dahlgren, M., Valeskog, K., Johansson, K., & Edelbring, S. (2022). Understanding clinical reasoning: a phenomenographic study with entry-level physiotherapy students. *Physiotherapy Theory and Practice, 38*(13), 2817–2826.

Andersson, C., & Törnberg, P. (2018). Wickedness and the anatomy of complexity. *Futures, 95*, 118–138.

Atkinson, H. L., & Nixon-Cave, K. (2011). A tool for clinical reasoning and reflection using the international classification of functioning, disability and health (ICF) framework and patient management model. *Physical Therapy, 91*(3), 416–430.

Bannigan, K., & Moores, A. (2009). A model of professional thinking: integrating reflective practice and evidence based practice. *Canadian Journal of Occupational Therapy, 76*(5), 342–350.

Benfield, A., & Jeffery, H. (2022). Exploring evidence based practice implementation by occupational therapists: implications for fieldwork. *Journal of Occupational Therapy Education, 6*(4), 10.

Blair, S. E. E., & Robertson, L. J. (2005). Hard complexities – soft complexities: an exploration of philosophical positions related to evidence in occupational therapy. *British Journal of Occupational Therapy, 68*(6), 269–276.

Bolton, T., & Dean, E. (2018). Self-determination theory and professional reasoning in occupational therapy students: a mixed methods study. *Journal of Occupational Therapy Education, 2*(3). https://doi.org/10.26681/jote.2018.020304

Botha, E. (2009). Why metaphor matters in education. *South African Journal of Education, 29*(4), 431–444.

Bransford, J. D., & Schwartz, D. L. (1999). Rethinking transfer: a simple proposal with multiple implications. *Review of Research in Education, 24*(61).

Broom, A., & Adams, J. (2012). A critical social science of evidence-based health care. In A. Broom & J. Adams (Eds.), *Evidence-based health care in context: Critical social science perspectives* (pp. 1–22). Ashgate Publishing Ltd.

Broom, A., & Tovey, P. (2012). Patient understandings of evidence and therapeutic effectiveness. In A. Broom & J. Adams (Eds.), *Evidence-based health care in context: Critical social science perspectives* (pp. 137–154). Ashgate Publishing Ltd.

Brynjolfsson, E., & McAfee, A. (2016). *The second machine age: Work, progress, and prosperity in a time of brilliant technologies.* W.W. Norton.

Buede, D. M., & Miller, W. D. (2016). *The engineering design of systems: Models and methods.* Wiley.

Christie, M., Carey, M., Robertson, A., & Grainger, P. (2015). Putting transformative learning theory into practice. *Australian Journal of Adult Learning, 55*(1), 9–30.

Clark, M. & Rossiter, M. (2008). Narrative Learning in the Adult Classroom. Adult Education Research Conference. https://newprairiepress.org/aerc/2008/papers/13

Dewey, J. (1910). *How we think.* D.C. Heath & Co.

Dewey, J. (1981). Experience is pedagogical: 26. My pedagogic creed. In J. J. McDermott (Ed.), *The philosophy of John Dewey: Two volumes in one* (pp. 442–454). University of Chicago Press.

Elstein, A., Shulman, L. S., & Sprafka, S. A. (1990). Medical problem solving: a ten-year retrospective. *Evaluation & the Health Professions, 13*(1), 5–39.

Endsley, M.R. (2001). Designing for situation awareness in complex system. Proceedings of the Second Intentional Workshop on Symbiosis of Humans, Artifacts and Environment.

Fish, D., & Coles, C. (1998). *Developing professional judgement in health care.* Heinemann.

Flynn, R., Greenhalgh, J., Long, A., & Tyson, S. (2012). Embodied, embedded and encoded knowledge in practice: the role of clinical interpretation in neurorehabilitation. In A. Broom & J. Adams (Eds.), *Evidence based health care in context: Critical social science perspectives* (pp. 77–96). Ashgate Publishing Ltd.

Gabbay, J., & le May, A. (2004). Evidence based guidelines or collectively constructed "mindlines?" Ethnographic study of knowledge management in primary care. *BMJ, 329*(7473), 1013.

Galbraith, K., Ward, A., & Heneghan, C. (2017). A real-world approach to evidence-based medicine in general practice: a competency framework derived from a systematic review and Delphi process. *BMC Medical Education, 17*(1), 1–15.

Gambrill, E. (2018). Contributions of the process of evidence-based practice to implementation: educational opportunities. *Journal of Social Work Education, 54*(suppl. 1), S113–S125.

Harrison, J.G. (2021). A developmental framework of practice for vocational and professional roles [Doctor of Philosophy, Victoria University]. https://vuir.vu.edu.au/42717/1/HARRISON_Jame-thesis_nosignature.pdf

Hoffman, T., Bennett, S., & Del Mar, C. (2017). Introduction to evidence-based practice. In T. Hoffman, S. Bennett, & C. Del Mar (Eds.), *Evidence-based practice across the health professions* (pp. 1–15). Elsevier Chatswood.

Innes, A. (2007). The consultation as a complex adaptive system. In J. Bogg & R. Geyer (Eds.), *Complexity science & society* (pp. 60–61). Radcliffe Publishing.

Jeffery, H., Robertson, L., & Reay, K. L. (2020). Sources of evidence for professional decision-making in novice occupational therapy practitioners: clinicians' perspectives. *British Journal of Occupational Therapy, 84*, 1–9.

Karbach, J. (1987). Using Toulmin's model of argumentation. *Journal of Teaching Writing, 6*(1), 81–92.

Kassirer, J., Wong, J., & Kopelman, R. (2010). *Learning clinical reasoning.* Wolters Kluwer/Lippincott Williams & Wilkins.

Klaic, M., McDermott, F., & Haines, T. (2018). How soon do allied health professionals lose confidence to perform EBP activities? A cross-sectional study. *Journal of Evaluation in Clinical Practice, 2018*, 603–612.

Klaic, M., McDermott, F., & Haines, T. (2019). Does the theory of planned behaviour explain allied health professionals' evidence-based practice behaviours? A focus group study. *Journal of Allied Health, 48*(1), e43–e51.

Klein, G., Snowden, D., & Pin, C. L. (2010). Anticipatory thinking. In K. L. Mosier & U. M. Fischer (Eds.), *Informed by knowledge: Expert performance in complex situations* (pp. 235–246). Psychology Press.

Knightbridge, L. (2019). Reflection-in-ractice: a survey of Australian occupational therapists. *Australian Occupational Therapy Journal, 66*(3), 337–346.

Lester, S. (1995). Beyond knowledge and competence. *Capability, 1*(3), 44–52.

Li, R. C., Smith, M., Lu, J., Avati, A., Wang, S., Teuteberg, W. G., Shum, K., Hong, G., Seevaratnam, B., Westphal, J., Dougherty, M., Rao, P., Asch, S., Lin, S., Sharp, C., Shieh, L., & Shah, N. H. (2022). Using AI to empower collaborative team workflows: two implementations for advance care planning and care escalation. *NEJM Catalyst, 3*(4), CAT.21.0457

Liaw, W., Kueper, J. K., Lin, S., Bazemore, A., & Kakadiaris, I. (2022). Competencies for the use of artificial intelligence in primary care. *Annals of Family Medicine, 20*(6), 559–563.

Mälkki, K. (2010). Building on Mezirow's theory of transformative learning: theorizing the challenges to reflection. *Journal of Transformative Education, 8*(1), 42–62.

Mankar, D., & Shaikh, D. A. (2021). Sociocultural perspectives of health. *Indian Practitioner, 74*, 7–9.

Markkanen, P., Välimäki, M., Anttila, M., & Kuuskorpi, M. (2020). A reflective cycle: understanding challenging situations in a school setting. *Educational Research, 62*(1), 46–62.

Mattingly, C. (1994). Clinical revision. In C. Mattingly & M. H. (. E.). Fleming (Eds.), *Clinical reasoning: Forms of inquiry in a therapeutic practice* (pp. 270–291). F.A. Davis.

Mezirow, J. (2018). Transformative learning theory. In K. Illeris (Ed.), *Contemporary theories of learning: Learning theorists . . . in their own words* (pp. 114–128). Routledge.

Monteiro, S., Sherbino, J., Sibbald, M., & Norman, G. (2020). Critical thinking, biases and dual processing: the enduring myth of generalisable skills. *Medical Education, 54*(1), 66–73.

Morin, E. (2008). *On complexity.* Hampton Press.

Pieris, D., Jafine, H., Neilson, S., Amster, E., Zazulak, J., Lam, C., & Grierson, L. (2022). Understanding moral empathy: a verbatim-theatre supported phenomenological exploration of the empathy imperative. *Medical Education, 56*(2), 186–194.

Pitama, S. G., Bennett, S. T., Waitoki, W., Haitana, T. N., Valentine, H., Pahina, J., Taylor, J. E., Tassell-Matamua, N., Rowe, L., Beckert, L., Palmer, S. C., Huria, T. M., Lacey, C. J., & McLachlan, A. (2017). A proposed Hauora Māori clinical guide for psychologists: using the Hui process and Meihana model in clinical assessment and formulation. *New Zealand Journal of Psychology, 46*(3), 7–19.

Ralston, P. A., & Bays, C. L. (2013). Enhancing critical thinking across the undergraduate experience: an exemplar from engineering. *American Journal of Engineering Education, 4*(2), 119–126.

Robertson, L., Graham, F., & Anderson, J. (2013). What actually informs practice: occupational therapists' views of evidence. *British Journal of Occupational Therapy, 76*(7), 317–324.

Rodgers, C. (2002). Defining reflection: another look at John Dewey and reflective thinking. *Teachers College Record, 104*(4), 842–866.

Rodgers, C. (2008). Leading change through informal coalitions. www.systemicleadershipinstitute.org/wp- content/uploads/2017/08/Leading- Change-Through Informal- Coalitions1.pdf

Rodrigues, S. M., Kanduri, A., Nyamati, A., Dut, N., Khargonekar, P., & Rhamani, A. M. (2022). Digital health-enabled community-centered care: scalable model to empower future community health workers using human-in-the-loop artificial intelligence. *JMIR Formative Research, 6*(4), e29535.

Rolfe, G., Jasper, M., & Freshwater, D. (2010). *Critical reflection in practice: Generating knowledge for care.* Red Globe Press.

Rycroft-Malone, J. (2004). The PARIHS framework – a framework for guiding the implementation of evidence-based practice. *Journal of Nursing Care Quality, 19*(4), 297–304.

Rycroft-Malone, J., Seers, K., Titchen, A., Harvey, G., Kitson, A., & McCormack, B. (2009). What counts as evidence in evidence based practice? *Journal of Advanced Nursing, 47*(1), 81–90.

Sackett, D. L., Rosenberg, W. M. C., Gray, M. J. A., & Haynes, R. B. (1996). Evidence based medicine: what it is and what it isn't. *British Medical Journal, 312*(7023), 71–72.

Schön, D. A. (1983). *The reflective practitioner: How professionals think in action.* Basic Books, Inc.

Schraw, G., Dunkle, M. E., & Bendixen, L. D. (1995). Cognitive process in well-defined and ill-defined problem solving. *Applied Cognitive Psychology, 9*, 523–538.

Sniderman, A. D., LaChapelle, K. J., Rachon, N. A., & Furberg, C. D. (2013). The necessity for clinical reasoning in the era of evidence-based medicine. *Mayo Clinic Proceedings, 88*(10), 1108–1114.

Snowden, D. J. (2000). The art and science of story or 'Are you sitting uncomfortably?': Part 1: Gathering and harvesting the raw material. *Business Information Review, 17*(3), 147–156.

Snyder, L. G., & Snyder, M. J. (2008). Teaching critical thinking and problem solving skills. *Delta Pi Epsilon Journal, 1*(2), 90–97.

Spring, B., Marchese, S. H., & Steglitz, J. (2019). History and process of evidence-based practice in mental health. In S. Dimidjian (Ed.), *Evidence-based practice in action: Bridging clinical science and intervention* (pp. 9–27). Guilford Press.

Taylor, E. W. (2014). Empathy: the stepchild of critical reflection and transformative learning. *Educational Reflective Practices, 2*, 5–22.

Thompson, B. (2012). Abductive reasoning and case formulation in complex cases. In L. Robertson (Ed.), *Clinical reasoning in occupational therapy: Controversies in practice* (pp. 15–30). Wiley Online Library.

Timmermans, S., & Angell, A. (2001). Evidence-based medicine, clinical uncertainty, and learning to doctor. *Journal of Health and Social Behavior, 42*(4), 342–359.

Tonelli, M. R., & Shapiro, D. (2020). Experiential knowledge in clinical medicine: use and justification. *Theoretical Medicine and Bioethics, 41*(2–3), 67–82.

Tonelli, M. R., & Upshur, R. E. G. (2019). A philosophical approach to addressing uncertainty in medical education. *Academic Medicine*, *94*(4), 507–511.

Turner, P. (2019). The ecology of healthcare. In P. Turner (Ed.), *Leadership in healthcare: Delivering organisational transformation and operational excellence* (pp. 17–43). Springer International Publishing.

Unsworth, C. A. (2018). Research and scholarship in clinical and professional reasoning. In B. A. B. Schell & J. W. Schell (Eds.), *Clinical and professional reasoning in occupational therapy*. Wolters Kluwer.

Van Woerkom, M., & Croon, M. (2008). Operationalising critically reflective work behaviour. *Personnel Review*, *37*(3), 317–331.

Voss, J. F., Fincher-Kiefer, R., Wiley, J., & Silfies, L. N. (1993). On the processing of arguments. *Argumentation*, *7*, 165–181.

Weick, K. E. (2012). Organized sensemaking: a commentary on processes of interpretive work. *Human Relations*, *65*(1), 141–153.

Weick, K. E., Sutcliffe, K. M., & Obstfeld, D. (2005). Organizing and the process of sense making. *Organization Science*, *16*(4), 409–421.

Whiteside, M., Smith, R., Gazarek, J., Bridge, F., & Shields, N. (2016). A framework for enabling evidence-based practice in allied health. *Australian Social Work*, *69*(4), 417–427.

Wieringa, S., & Greenhalgh, T. (2015). 10 years of mindlines: a systematic review and commentary. *Implementation Science*, *10*(1), 45.

Woermann, M., & Cilliers, P. (2012). The ethics of complexity and the complexity of ethics. *South African Journal of Philosophy*, *31*(2), 447–463.

Zhang, S., & Li, H. (2022). The construction of an action-speech feature-based school violence recognition algorithm and occupational therapy education model for adolescents. *Occupational Therapy International*, *2022*, 1723736.

CHAPTER 3

Grasping the Whole: The Practitioner Perspective

Practitioner Influences on Professional Decisions

Sian E. Griffiths[1], Kim Reay[2], and Helen Jeffery[3]

[1]Principal Lecturer, School of Occupational Therapy, Te Pūkenga|Otago Polytechnic, New Zealand

[2]Lecturer, Occupational Therapy Department, Auckland University of Technology, New Zealand

[3]Principal Lecturer, School of Occupational Therapy, Te Pūkenga|Otago Polytechnic, New Zealand

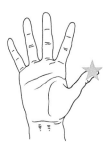

INTRODUCTION

The Five Finger Framework (FFF) forms a complex reasoning framework of which the practitioner is a component, represented on the framework by the thumb. How information and experience are managed by the practitioner profoundly influences the meaning that is constructed and decisions arrived at. As a fit between the situation and existing knowledge, values, and beliefs is constructed, our unique way of practicing emerges and what we choose to do in each situation evolves.

In using the analogy of a hand to depict professional reasoning, having the thumb represent the practitioner (self) is intentional. One of the most important movements of the hand is the thumb's opposition to the fingers. Opposition is a combination of several movements which allows the thumb and fingers to come together; this movement of opposition is fundamental for grasping and manipulating objects. The opposition of the thumb with the fingers creates a range of movements which

Professional Reasoning in Healthcare: Navigating Uncertainty Using the Five Finger Framework, First Edition.
Edited by Helen Jeffery, Linda Robertson, Jan Hendrik Roodt, and Susan Ryan.
© 2024 John Wiley & Sons Ltd. Published 2024 by John Wiley & Sons Ltd.

are greater and more complicated than the simple sum of the individual joints and, in turn, elicit skilled and coordinated functions of the hand. Indeed, opposition and the movement of the thumb has been said to be a crucial element of human civilization.

In the same way that the thumb can move in opposition to the fingers and be an integral part of the whole range of hand functions, so can the practitioner be an integral part in eliciting detailed and relevant information from all four other sources of information identified in the FFF. And in the same way that the thumb's interaction with the fingers can change a grip, so too can the practitioner, in their interaction with all the components, influence that information. Each piece of information, when drawn together, interacts with another to change the overall significance and ultimately the overall picture as it is viewed from the practitioner's perspective.

It is the practitioner's accessing information from the other four domains in combination with their unique reasoning that creates synergy, where the sum of the understanding and knowledge from the individual components results in professional decisions unique to the practitioner (Jeffery et al., 2021). The joints of the thumb have planes of movement to enable a wide range and variety of movements. When a specific pattern of movement is required in the thumb, the body enables only the elements required for that movement. So too can the practitioner become highly skilled in their reasoning about what, how, and how much they choose to interact with the four other sources of information – other professionals, clients, contextual factors, and their engagement with literature.

This process demands critical consideration of complex factors. Understanding the pragmatic demands of the workplace requirements, the unfolding narrative of the client, underpinning scientific knowledge held by the practitioner, and

the shared experience between client and practitioner in the moment all influence decisions about the pathway to follow and action to take. This requires skill in breaking the whole down into parts and appreciating the value of each part in the process (analysis), selecting what is most important, and deliberately considering those parts so that a new whole is created and informs an understanding unique to the situation (synthesis). Judgment regarding what holds value in the professional reasoning process occurs before, during, and after each client interaction, this evaluation guiding not only practice in the moment but changes to future practice decisions. In addition to these critical thinking skills, self-awareness (an awareness of who we are and our unique cultural influences and biases), conscious use of self, capacity to learn from others and respond to feedback all contribute to maintaining lifelong professional development.

Setting the Scene

I am an occupational therapist working in a busy city-based pediatric service. We offer assessment and intervention in the clinic, and to a lesser extent in the client's home when appropriate. I have over six years' experience working in pediatrics. Over the last three years, I have worked predominantly with children who have developmental difficulties, and with their families. I work as part of a multidisciplinary team with a focus on pediatric rehabilitation and management of complex conditions; the team advocates and provides support for families and caregivers and creates an environment that facilitates this. In particular, the children I work with have difficulty with coordination and movement-related function, developmental delay, and cognitive function which affects performance skills such as sitting, gross motor skills, fine motor skills, process (cognitive) skills, and self-help skills.

Jack is a three-year-old boy who lives with his mother, father, and two siblings – he has a five-year-old brother and a sister who is 16 months old. Jack has cerebral palsy.

I have used the FFF previously to help my understanding of what I bring to each experience and how the framework supports my clinical reasoning. I feel comfortable using this framework and know that several of my colleagues are also familiar with it.

The FFF provides cues for reflection (in action and on action), ensuring there is breadth of what is reflected on and depth in terms of insight gained from the reflection. Importantly, the FFF is also a useful tool for use in supervision and can provide structure for both the supervisor and the supervisee when grappling with inevitable complexity in practice.

Jack is one of five new pediatric referrals that have come into the team today. Mondays are designated for the assessment of new referrals and so are busy. I know I need to work quickly to get through my share of the work, but my knowledge and experience of pediatric clients have developed over time and so I feel confident I will complete a good assessment. I ascertained from the notes that Jack has been assessed previously by health professionals external to this team. He has developmental delay and has not reached milestones within the expected timeframes. Jack had seen a pediatrician and a rehab physician within a local hospital and was referred to us for multiple factors relating to motor, information processing, and social functioning. The referral was for a multidisciplinary team approach. After his appointment with me, he would be seen by other members of this team.

PROFESSIONAL KNOWLEDGE AND IDENTITY

All these appointments can be a test of stamina for clients as information is gathered by multidisciplinary team members. Although this can seem repetitive for the client, I can see the benefits of having a team approach to ensure Jack, his family, staff, and the organization see valued therapeutic outcomes (Nancarrow et al., 2013). Interdisciplinary practice requires me to hold an awareness of the role of others in the team as well as my own expertise and guides my decisions regarding what information I will gather from Jack and his family, what I will look for in the documentation, and what is less important for me to know. This comes easily to me now as I have a well-established professional identity which enables me to focus on information pertinent to my professional discipline, and I appreciate the specific focus professionals from other disciplines in the team will have. Maintaining and adapting one's professional identity requires shared ontology, embracing the culture of the profession, enacting the profession, and believing in the profession (Walder et al., 2022). These factors guide us in terms of how to think, act, and feel in terms of professional identity. I can see that the way that I think, act, and feel both influences and is influenced by my professional identity, and so guides my work within the team.

Teamwork is significant in terms of improving the client experience (Best et al., 2021), and the interdisciplinary team I am a part of values teamwork and collaboration. Through discussions with other team members, I understand the differences in professional perspectives the team draws from to support clients to achieve their goals. Collaborative team working in this way enhances overall professional reasoning – by both ensuring that the client (client finger) is central and tapping into the expertise of the team, valuable knowledge, and skills are drawn on ensuring the process results in a quality outcome for both the client and the organization (Olson et al., 2020).

I am grateful for the opportunities I have within my team for collaboration, knowing that this is helpful for professional reasoning (Taylor, 2020). Sharing challenges and celebrations with the team is an effective form of informal supervision that helps to clarify our thinking, particularly when we take the time to share our reasoning processes with each other. I remember as a novice practitioner I wanted to know everything, believing that this was the way to develop. But keeping up with all the knowledge was overwhelming, and I learned to look for patterns and cues, work with the knowledge of the client and family, and learn from peers and experiences, which was more realistic. I do find that interacting with my peers helps me work out how I am thinking, and differences of opinion trigger me to think more critically about my work. This has sometimes resulted in me solidifying my position and at other times led to me making a change to my practice.

As part of my preparation for this initial assessment, I thought about how I like to work, and the way that I now use the knowledge I have. Of course, I have gained a lot of what is sometimes referred to as propositional knowledge – this is the knowledge that relates to facts and principles such as anatomy and lifespan development, important when working with children (Schell & Benfield, 2018).

My decision to work with Jack on his reach and grasp using his upper limbs is supported by this form of knowledge (research and literature finger). Much of this was through my initial training and subsequent formal educational opportunities. I do try and keep up with advances in the field of occupational therapy and pediatrics, but this is sometimes difficult. I often feel grateful for our leadership team who review overall literature annually and ensure our protocols reflect current best practice. I know that Jack and his family as well as my team members all have expectations of my role and of me as a member of the team. The knowledge I hold and how I choose to use it will be important for the overall process.

On reading pertinent notes on the file in preparation for the initial interviewm I was able to quickly build up a picture of Jack, how he might present, and what I might do with him today. I remember the days when the file review would take me much longer, and I would still feel poorly prepared – I reflected on this and just how much knowledge I hold. It feels like common sense now, but I know this is what Mattingly and Fleming (1994) identify as the use of tacit knowledge. This is a type of knowledge that is acquired through lived professional experience and includes wisdom, intuition, and insights into the situation based on previous experiences. Tacit knowledge is often at an almost subconscious level and is accessed automatically rather than in a focused cognitive process. It builds up over time as propositional knowledge and active experiences are embedded in the self and enables practitioners to work increasingly efficiently as they acquire the ability to act almost automatically (Mattingly & Fleming, 2019).

This knowledge developed from previous experience of working with children with physical and developmental difficulties and their families and has become integrated with everything else I know.

I am confident in completing assessments and developing plans with my clients that fit around their life and their needs; this is not something that I could have said at the start of my work in pediatrics. Many of my skills have been honed through experience. Experiential learning is defined as a particular way of learning through engaging in activity, reflecting on what happened, making meaning from the insights gained through reflection, and acting on those insights (Kolb, 2015). I remember the fieldwork education placements that formed a part of my undergraduate education – these were so powerful for me as I saw theory being implemented, saw practitioners challenge ideas, and adapt theory to fit their practice context. I developed an understanding of the importance of emotions in everyday interactions between therapists and clients, and, most importantly, I was able to practice skills myself. This not only helped me consolidate knowledge and skills but enabled me to work out a picture of who I was in my professional role, and the personal traits and strengths I have that are helpful in my work.

Experiences I have at work continue to build my knowledge base and practice style, and use of frameworks such as Kolb's (2015) experiential learning cycle in supervision continues to help me consolidate that learning in a way that benefits my future practice.

EMOTIONAL INTELLIGENCE

As part of preparation for our initial meeting, I considered the question "Who is my client?" I knew details of Jack but little of his family. As he is a child, the family are as much the client as he is. From Jack's file, I ascertained that Jack and his family had been waiting for pediatric community services for just over a year and had very little in the way of support at home. I felt empathetic – not only was life difficult for the family but professional support services were likely limited. Empathy, the capacity to both understand and experience the feelings of another person (Preston & de Waal, 2002), is part of holistic communication that although complex can have a powerful influence in building effective collaborative relationships with clients. O'Toole (2020) identifies that empathy can be verbal and nonverbal expression but requires the person working with the client to listen and understand what the client is feeling in a nonjudgmental way. Thus, empathy is an emotional response that helps the practitioner view the client's situation and respond in a way that demonstrates care, support, and understanding and is a way of using emotional intelligence (Mayer & Cobb, 2000) in practice.

Empathy, as with any emotion, emerges or is triggered within us but can be developed or enhanced over time. I have learned that for myself understanding a client's situation, using what I know in terms of the health challenge and thinking holistically has resulted in my capacity to experience empathy. Being able to express this has been helpful in terms of enhancing therapeutic relationships. As I tried to put myself in their situation and thought about the frustration and emotions that can naturally manifest, I realized I needed to acknowledge this when I met Jack and his family – this awareness of and preparedness to work with the emotions of self and the other is important when working in healthcare (Taylor et al., 2009). Finding the appropriate demeanor that is warm, friendly, and empathetic would be crucial. Effective skills in managing emotions that arise is important for collaboration, optimism, and engagement that can then help foster a particular client–practitioner relationship, an intentional relationship (Taylor, 2020).

I started to plan the assessment session and what I could bring to the initial meeting with the family. As well as empathy, I am aware of my other personal qualities and strengths, including interpersonal skills such as communication and listening, my pragmatic approach to problem solving, and my gentle sense of humor. I am aware of how these traits can encourage parents or caregivers to feel at ease with me and share their narrative. My level of self-awareness has increased over the years and been enhanced through intentional reflection and use of supervision. Self-awareness, or being conscious of who we are including our values and beliefs, underpins our capacity to be reflective and to consciously use ourselves in therapeutic interactions (Bulman & Schutz, 2013). This concept also involves awareness of what we are feeling, how we are responding to feelings, and what we are portraying to others. Introspection, or evaluating our practice to make decisions or ascertain how we are doing, demands awareness of ourselves – ultimately, the way we process and come to understand our inner world influences what we say and do in the "outside world" – our practice (Atkins & Schultz, 2013; Ekroth-Bucher, 2010). As I compare how I work now with when I was a newly graduated practitioner, I recognize just how much more aware I am of the role of my "self" in my practice, and of the importance of continuing to develop and maintain awareness of myself.

The initial meeting was scheduled to take place in the clinic with follow-up appointments over the next two weeks either in the clinic or at the family's home. Having heard the noises of people approaching in the corridor, I quickly went over in my mind what I knew from the referral and checked that I had prepared well for the session. I checked that the environment was suitable for Jack to engage in play. The play mat was on the floor, the toys were laid out

ready, a selection of brightly colored blocks, stacking toys, and a peg board that I hoped would attract Jack's attention and allow me to assess him as he played with them. His 16-month-old sister was joining us, and I arranged the room to be safe for both. I put the file in the drawer of my table, I checked Jack's mother's and sister's names, making a mental note to remember them. As I walked over to the door, I could hear bumping sounds from the corridor. I wondered again why we must have such doors; they are heavy for anyone but impossible to manage with a buggy. I imagined the frustration of his mother, whose name is Mia, trying to navigate certain environments and I wondered whether the home environment presented such challenges, making a note to check this with them.

Mia, as expected, was struggling with the door and a twin buggy, which both children were strapped in, the hood of the buggy laden with coats, bags, toys, and topped off with a small pink cardigan. Mia was having a problem keeping all their belongings from falling to the floor whilst trying to lean to push the door open. As I held the door open, Mia smiled at me and I smiled back, but I felt embarrassed, thinking, "What sort of first impression does it make when the doors in the corridor outside my office are inappropriate?" Moreover, I felt annoyed as I remembered the reasons I was given as to why they could not be changed. I was expected to advise on access and adaptation, provide a welcoming environment, and I could not even get suitable doors in the corridor outside my room. I examined the way I was feeling and the cause of this. I wanted to create a good first impression when meeting Jack and his family and I felt frustrated that could not be achieved. It was important to me that I showed to the family that I was a competent professional. I was also very aware that Jack and his mother would both be weighing up the situation and me – how they felt toward me would also influence how our relationship developed and how the therapeutic process unfolded. This would be as crucial as the formal assessments and therapy I provided.

The range of feelings I was experiencing in this initial meeting with Jack and his family, even before meeting them, was likely to influence my interactions and professional reasoning. I had rapid shifts from one emotion to another as I discarded the frustration I was feeling, which had begun with the inability of my client to access the department and included my understanding of institutional challenges which had caused a long wait time for an assessment for Jack. Professionals are not isolated from their emotions; it is the acquiring and applying of knowledge and skills so that an individual is able to manage and make use of such emotions when they arise that is important. I have grown as a clinician with the ability to recognize emotions and become more aware of the impact varying emotions can have on my relationship with my clients and the way I think and practice, an element of emotional intelligence. McKenna and Mellson (2013) acknowledge that the ability to manage emotions can affect the practitioner's effectiveness and conclude that the value placed on emotional intelligence is key to practice.

Emotional intelligence is a domain of study from psychology and is proposed to be a facet of overall intelligence. It is defined by Andonian (2017) as "An ability to monitor feelings and emotions and to use the information to guide thinking and problem solving" (p. 300). Emotional intelligence requires the four skills of perceiving emotions in self and others, using emotional information to inform communication or thinking, understanding emotions, and managing emotions (Andonian, 2017; Mayer et al., 2002, 2004). These skills can be measured in the Mayer Salovey Caruso Emotional Intelligence Test (Mayer et al., 2002), which explores ability in emotional intelligence. I had completed this test some years ago which made me much more aware of the place of emotion in professional reasoning and practice. Ongoing reflection has developed my skills in using my emotional knowledge and abilities. In this initial meeting, I gathered myself, took a deep breath and focused on being mindfully present as I welcomed the family into the room.

Ten minutes later and I am on the floor with Jack and his sister. From my initial observation of Jack playing with some of the toys and listening to Mia, I could tell that my involvement with Jack and his family would be long term. I was able to form a view of this family that drew from all my knowledge and reasoning processes. Known as conditional reasoning, this is the capacity not just to appreciate where the client is in the moment but to envisage a possible future (Fleming, 1991), which is helpful in terms of holistic thinking and planning and scaffolding interventions (Schell & Benfield, 2018). The use of conditional reasoning can help with intervention planning with Jack and Mia but I need to be careful not to overly anticipate what the future might look like – appreciating likely trajectories and holding hope for positive outcomes is a benefit of conditional reasoning. This awareness must be tempered with ongoing analysis of the present, what is working and what is not. I continued with my assessment, using play as a vehicle to assess Jack whilst at the same time asking Mia questions and observing the interaction between Jack and his sister.

THERAPEUTIC USE OF SELF

As practitioners, we adapt our use of self to how we respond to each therapeutic encounter and recognize how this is essential to the way we practice. This is sometimes known as the therapeutic use of self, which Punwar and Peloquin (2000) describe as ". . .a practitioner's planned use of his or her personality, insights, perceptions, and judgments, as part of the therapeutic process" (p. 285). Therapeutic use of self is in part informed by emotional intelligence and is expressed through relational skills (Andonian, 2017).

I placed myself on the floor opposite Jack to play at his level. I expressed empathy and support to Mia as she talked through challenges that she was experiencing but changed to a more light-hearted tone to engage Jack and encourage him to continue to play. Using elements of self and using play, I can assess several performance components including observing movement, cognition, and the social connectedness to his sister and mother. Importantly, I am using my self to guide many elements of this process in a way that is effective for them and feels comfortable to me.

Later in the assessment, Jack had stopped playing with the toys and his sister was now asleep in the pram. I sat on the floor with Jack, encouraging different elements of play that I had not observed when he was with his sister. I started to talk with his mother about Jack's social environment such as his play friends, places they may go, and what they like to do. She started to become reticent about sharing information and this progressed to her becoming very distressed, she burst into tears and found it very difficult to talk with me. This resulted in me feeling uncertain about how to cope, as her level of emotion had shifted so dramatically that it took me by surprise. I intentionally used a calm and soothing tone to help her regulate her emotions. The emotions experienced during an interaction between two or more people are cocreated on a moment-by-moment basis. This is sometimes named coregulation and can be used intentionally

where one's response to another's distress is helpful for their emotional expression and/or regulation. Despite my best efforts, Mia remained distressed and stated that she really needed to go. They left quickly without me really understanding what had caused the distress. I continued to feel uncomfortable myself, an example of the client's emotional state affecting my own (Guendelman et al., 2022).

Following the session with Jack and his family, I needed to take time to work out what had happened. Professional reasoning is in part based on complex interactions between people and their environments – this certainly turned out to be a complex situation for me. Chapparo and Ranka (2019) propose six questions that form the "heart" of occupational therapy assessment and intervention.

- What is the situation?
- What is wanted/needed/possible in this situation?
- What will I do?
- How will I do it?
- Why am I doing it?
- Did it work?

I understood what I chose to take into consideration and my interpretation of that information would inform me of my next move.

REFLECTIVE PRACTICE

Reflection plays an important role in helping me make sense of and learn from experience, is often triggered by a strong emotional response, and is helpful in processing and making sense of these emotional experiences. Reflection is complex and to be of benefit requires time and attention. In supervision, I am encouraged to use reflection for processing experiences and learning, and to use a tool to guide the reflection – I often use Kolb and Kolb's reflective cycle (2018) or Fish et al.'s (1991) Strands model, as well as the FFF to help me integrate my learning through reflection with my overall professional reasoning.

This time, the uncomfortable feelings I was left with motivated me to try and work it out carefully. I wanted to question the impact of what happened, consider any alternative action I could have taken, and identify what I could do differently in the future (Jasper, 2003). It was important for me to learn from this experience in a way that would inform my next interaction with Mia and deepen my understanding of their situation, and of our relationship. This focus on learning for myself and the potential implications of the interaction on our future work together is an example of critical thinking.

I decided to use the Fish et al. reflection model (1991), also known as "Strands," as I had used this previously and found it helpful. Strands refers to four aspects of a reflective experience to help with developing a depth of understanding. The four threads of practice are explained by Fish (2012) as: the *factual* strand in which I describe the event, the *retrospective* strand in which I look back over the whole event and identify key patterns or elements of the experience that stand out, the *substratum* strand that enables me to reflect on my personal theory linked to values, beliefs, and assumptions. These three strands are drawn together to form the fourth, the *connective* strand, which enables me to identify my learning from this, what further formal learning I might need to do, and how I might do things differently in the future. I completed a written reflection using the four Strands, so that I could be well prepared for supervision the following week.

Writing notes as I moved through the strands of reflection proved to be thought-provoking, and the connection that I made in the fourth strand was insightful. I realized that I had assumed (based on my own

experience of family life and that of many of my previous clients) that the family would be able to or want to participate in social events or outings. I had rushed into aspects of the assessment without finding out more about them as a family and what was important to them. My focus during most of the session was on ascertaining the functional problems as I worked through my assessment tool and working out potential solutions. This is referred to by Mattingly and Fleming (1994) as procedural reasoning, where the emphasis is on maximizing a client's functioning. The focus of my thinking (and consequently questioning and actions) was on problem solving, I had omitted to consider what was front of mind for Jack and his family and had not maintained a holistic or family-centered approach. It dawned on me that this unconscious bias was in part caused by my use of tacit knowledge and the routines I had formed for initial assessment, as well as my assumptions regarding the social habits and needs of people.

SUPERVISION

In the supervision session, I took along my written reflection and my motivation to critically explore this incident. Workloads and time pressures can affect formal reflection in practice (Knightbridge, 2019), I really wanted to make the most of my precious hour of supervision. My supervisor follows a model of supervision which feels safe and guides us through the session so that ethics and processes are explored, there is a plan for the session, and a sense of completion by the end. This requires me to come prepared with a topic or issue and a desired outcome that we agree to work toward.

Supervision is central to my professional development and provides a safe space and time for me to reflect on my caseload and any ethical incidents or dilemmas that may have arisen. For me to learn from supervision, I am aware of my responsibility to be transparent and honest when exploring what I have brought to focus on, and I trust that my supervisor will act with equal integrity and honesty (Feasy, 2002). I had already considered that my questioning about social elements of the family's life might have been based on an unconscious bias, but that equally it could be a legitimate element of overall psychosocial assessment and could have triggered an emotional response from Mia because of underlying social issues.

My supervisor had a rough drawing of a hand on the table so that we could check in on the fingers of the FFF as they arose, and I had my written reflection with me. I began with the "factual strand" to set the scene and the key moments as they happened. This strand needed unpicking as I identified the incident and pinpointed conversation and actions leading up to the point where Jack's mother became distressed and left. I moved onto the "retrospective" strand, and looked back over the whole event, I reflected on what was my aim for this session, and what were the successes and failures. With prompting from my supervisor, I recognized that interactions with Jack and his mother seemed to be going well from my perspective. I was observing and noting what I needed to about Jack's skills in play and communication with me, and I had allowed his mother to talk through the challenges and issues at home. She had answered my questions openly, which I thought was evidence of a collaborative relationship. I am confident my communication skills are strong, that in this instance I had related appropriately and had conveyed empathy and care. So what had triggered the distress and forced such an abrupt end to the session? My supervisor pointed to the client finger on the drawn hand and encouraged me to try and explore new meanings of the incident through analyzing it from the viewpoint of the client. I moved onto what is named the substratum

strand of this model to explore assumptions I had made, actions in the session or beliefs that had influenced my interactions and contributed to Mia's distress.

Here I struggled. Each time I was nudged to view the session through the client's eyes, I could not see a reason for distress, and I found myself feeling challenged and defensive. My supervisor explained that I had provided a good summary of the situation and what is required in the initial assessment from my perspective, and my rationale for the assessments chosen was appropriate. He asks me to focus more on the question "why" did I structure the session that way, and "why" did I ask the questions I did. From my perspective, my rationale was sound but again he pointed to the client finger on the hand. He then gently asked me if I was in a space to be able to hear some feedback from him. Of course, I said "yes," I felt I needed to be seen to be a good supervisee as much as I wanted to be seen as a good therapist (an attitude I was to learn was influential in my professional reasoning).

As he talked about his perspective of how I have developed my professional reasoning style, it became clear I was using procedural reasoning (with a very strong focus on problem identification and functional solutions) and that pragmatic reasoning was also evident through my wanting to make the most of the hour-long session that was scheduled for Jack, my need to fill in the paperwork at the end of the session and have a plan for therapy to feed back to the team at our next meeting. Why I asked the questions I did was driven by what needed to be documented, and my need to be an effective problem solver and solution-focused practitioner, so in many respects I was preempting the outcome of the session. I had involved Mia in the discussion to have her respond to my ideas and in doing so I had not collaborated on anything, and I had managed and controlled the conversation to remain in the area that I felt confident I could address. The only time Mia was able to take any control was when she cried and left the session.

We talked through the reasons why this might be happening; some of it was pragmatic – I needed to get that assessment done! However, a legitimate part of the assessment is the family perspective of priorities and needs, and this was missed through my reluctance to allow Mia to have some control of the conversation. Was this just about time pressure or was this a lack of confidence in being able to deal with what might be raised? Or a focus on my personal beliefs about who I "should be" in this role and the expectation of others on me? Or was there some arrogance in my stance – I had so much experience in pediatrics, I thought I already knew what I needed to do with this family. My perception of what I was there to do, whilst accurate, was a limiting factor in my reasoning and in my formation of a genuine relationship with Jack and his mother. I could not come to any conclusion about the reason for the distress as I had not enabled her to share enough of her perspective and the overall family situation.

Although I felt vulnerable and a little upset, my supervisor helped me appreciate what had happened through describing the Johari Window model (Luft & Ingham, 1961). This model of self-awareness has four quadrants.

- Open area (known to others and to self)
- Blind spot (known to others, not known to self)
- Hidden area (not known to others, known to self)
- Unknown (not known to others, not known to self)

This supervision session was a lightbulb moment for me, as something about me that was known to my supervisor but unknown to me was revealed.

This experience and the consequent supervision session also illustrated my tendency to touch base with the literature finger (with my established routines in evidence-based practice) and the context finger in terms of following policies and workplace procedures. I utilize the expertise of others through my engagement in wider pediatric communities and attendance at conferences. However, despite believing I had focused on the client's perspective, I had been doing this at a very superficial level. Perhaps being more transparent about my thoughts and plans with Mia as I formed them may have allowed us to reason together. I have enough experience to be able to relinquish some control and cope with any complexity that might emerge – I resolved to ascertain and use the expertise of the client, and to genuinely collaborate with the client going forward. I am learning to change myself to be the practitioner the client needs in the moment through becoming an expert in myself as well as in my professional work.

Returning to the analogy of a hand to depict professional reasoning, having the thumb represent the practitioner (self) requires constant awareness of the influence of the practitioner on professional reasoning. I must recognize that I am the one who is doing the reasoning and the one who will be writing the report, making recommendations, accessing funding, and deciding on or implementing a course of action. While I am often not the person who makes the ultimate decision, I am the link between a client and those who do. So, the balance of power between myself and other components is very much in my favor. Like the interaction between the thumb and the fingers in opposition for the manipulation of objects, I am the person who has the greatest ability to manipulate all the other sources of evidence, either intentionally or unconsciously. This power is precious and must be used ethically and with care.

As I explore the sources of evidence, I can discover new things or choose to only explore what I already know. In the scenario with Jack, I was only exploring what I knew and therefore more likely to feel safe and able to manage the situation or issues that arose. In carefully planning and managing the assessment, I was very likely to find out what I needed to know to answer the questions that I had. I was also therefore likely to be able to demonstrate the knowledge that I had to Jack and his family, or to my colleagues in my report. However, I was far less likely to learn any more than I already knew, or thought I needed to know, about Jack and his family or about my own development as an occupational therapist. It was Jack's mother's refusal to follow my plan that provided me with a very important learning experience.

Looking at the FFF, I am reminded to gather information, or evidence, from many areas and synthesize it so that it fits together as new knowledge about a particular client, in a particular situation. This synthesis, the fitting together of the information, is my knowledge translation (Strauss et al., 2009) and is my professional reasoning (Figure 3.1).

SUMMARY

This chapter has focused on how influential the "self" is, how we use our selves to influence professional reasoning and therefore client outcomes. Reference has been made to how crucial it is to regularly touch base with the other fingers to maintain the strength and flexibility of the thumb. The key points of this chapter are summarized in Table 3.1.

Tools in Chapter 9 provide ideas on how to focus on self in reasoning, and the reflection tools may be of particular interest.

The next chapter illustrates the role of the index finger in pointing to the value of drawing on the expertise of others in professional reasoning.

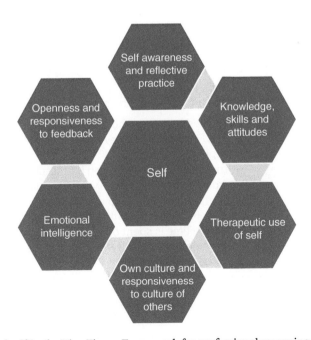

FIGURE 3.1   Use of self in the Five Finger Framework for professional reasoning.

TABLE 3.1   Key Points

Role	Key Points
Practitioner/ student	• Learn about and prepare for supervision. • Use a reflection model. • Use a variety of techniques to stimulate reflection. • Practice conscious therapeutic use of self. • Enhance emotional intelligence through reflection, supervision, and intentional learning. • Use experiential learning intentionally.
Educator	• Include learning about what supervision is and how to best use it. • Include interdisciplinary practice education. • Emphasize what is unique about the profession to initiate professional identity – the knowledge, skills, values, culture, and practices specific to the profession. • Teach reflective practice and a model of reflection. • Explore reflection techniques and triggers with learners. • Use experiential learning. • Enhance teamwork skills through team projects/activities. • Individual values and professional values. • Teach therapeutic use of self.
Manager	• Provide ongoing education opportunities to increase propositional knowledge in staff. • Enable practice observations between novice and experienced practitioners. • Enable supervision. • Have trustworthy evidence-based protocols and processes. • Enable and nurture profession-specific practice and culture to strengthen professional identity. • Nurture interprofessional collaboration and opportunities for teamworking. • Provide opportunities for staff to share professional reasoning. • Use group or team reflection strategies.
Supervisor	• Utilize supervision model or structure. • Use Five Finger Framework to ensure breadth and enable depth to supervision. • Trigger/stimulate reflection in the supervisee. • Frame supervision as a way of building the strength of the thumb in the Five Finger Framework. • Explore reasoning with supervisee. • Ensure time is spent on emotions, therapeutic use of self and relationships between supervisee and client. • Focus on ethics.

REFERENCES

Andonian, L. (2017). Emotional intelligence: an opportunity for occupational therapy. *Occupational Therapy in Mental Health, 33*(4), 299–307.

Atkins, S., & Schultz, S. (2013). Developing skills for reflective practice. In C. Bulman & S. Schutz (Eds.), *Reflective practice in nursing* (pp. 23–52). John Wiley & Sons.

Best, S., Beech, C., Robbe, I. J., & Williams, S. (2021). Interprofessional teamwork: the role of professional identity and signature pedagogy – a mixed methods study. *Journal of Health Organization and Management, 35*(5), 561–578.

Bulman, C., & Schutz, S. (2013). *Reflective practice in nursing* (5th ed.). John Wiley & Sons.

Chapparo, C., & Ranka, J. (2019). Clinical reasoning in occupational therapy. In J. Higgs, G. M. Jensen, S. Loftus, & N. Christensen (Eds.), *Clinical reasoning in the health professions* (pp. 271–283). Elsevier Ltd.

Ekroth-Bucher, M. (2010). Self-awareness: a review and analysis of a basic nursing concept. *Advances in Nursing Science, 33*(4), 297–309.

Feasy, D. (2002). *Good practice in supervision with psychotherapists and counsellors: A relational approach.* Wiley.

Fish, D. (2012). Strands to the invisibles: from a technical to a moral mode of reflective practice. In G. Boniface & A. Seymour (Eds.), *Using occupational therapy theory in practice* (pp. 38–48). John Wiley & Sons.

Fish, D., Twinn, S., & Purr, B. (1991). *Promoting reflection: Improving the supervision of practice in health visiting and initial teacher training.* West London Institute.

Fleming, M. H. (1991). The therapist with the three-track mind. *American Journal of Occupational Therapy, 45*(11), 988–996.

Guendelman, S., Bayer, M., Prehn, K., & Dziobek, I. (2022). Regulating negative emotions of others reduces own stress: neurobiological correlates and the role of individual differences in empathy. *NeuroImage, 254*, 119134.

Jasper, M. (2003). *Beginning reflective practice.* Nelson Thorne.

Jeffery, H., Robertson, L., & Reay, K. L. (2021). Sources of evidence for professional decision-making in novice occupational therapy practitioners: clinicians' perspectives. *British Journal of Occupational Therapy, 84*(6), 346–354.

Knightbridge, L. (2019). Reflection-in-practice: a survey of Australian occupational therapists. *Australian Occupational Therapy Journal, 66*, 337–346.

Kolb, A., & Kolb, D. (2018). Eight important things to know about the experiential learning cycle. *Australian Educational Leader, 40*(3), 8–14.

Kolb, D. (2015). *Experiential learning: Experience as the source of learning and development* (2nd ed.). Pearson Education.

Luft, J., & Ingham, H. (1961). The Johari window. *Human Relations Training News, 5*(1), 6–7.

Mattingly, C., & Fleming, M. H. (1994). *Clinical reasoning: Forms of inquiry in a therapeutic practice.* F.A. Davis.

Mattingly, C., & Fleming, M. H. (2019). Action and narrative: two dynamics of clinical reasoning. In J. Higgs, G. M. Jensen, S. Loftus, & N. Christensen (Eds.), *Clinical reasoning in the health professions* (pp. 119–127). Elsevier Health Sciences.

Mayer, J. D., & Cobb, C. D. (2000). Educational policy on emotional intelligence – does it make sense? *Educational Psychology Review, 12*(2), 163–183.

Mayer, J. D., Salovey, P., & Caruso, D. (2002). *Mayer-Salovey-Caruso Emotional Intelligence Test (MSCEIT) user's manual.* Multi-Health Systems Inc.

Mayer, J. D., Salovey, P., & Caruso, D. (2004). Emotional intelligence: theory, findings, and implications. *Psychological Inquiry*, *15*(3), 197–215.

McKenna, J., & Mellson, A. (2013). Emotional intelligence and the occupational therapist. *British Journal of Occupational Therapy*, *76*(9), 76–79.

Nancarrow, S. A., Booth, A., Ariss, S., Smith, T., Enderby, P., & Roots, A. (2013). Ten principles of good interdisciplinary team work. *Human Resources for Health*, *11*, 19.

Olson, A. P. J., Durning, S. J., Fernandez Branson, C., Sick, B., Lane, K. P., & Rencic, J. J. (2020). Teamwork in clinical reasoning – cooperative or parallel play. *Diagnosis*, *7*(3), 307–312.

O'Toole, G. (2020). *Communication. Core interpersonal skills for healthcare professionals* (4th ed.). Elsevier.

Preston, S. D., & De Waal, F. B. (2002). Empathy: its ultimate and proximate bases. *Behavioral and Brain Sciences*, *25*(1), 1–20.

Punwar, A. J., & Peloquin, S. M. (2000). *Occupational therapy: Principles and practice* (3rd ed.). Lippincott, Williams & Wilkins.

Schell, B. A. B., & Benfield, A. (2018). Aspects of professional reasoning. In B. A. B. Schell & J. Schell (Eds.), *Clinical and professional reasoning in occupational therapy* (pp. 127–144). Wolters Kluwer.

Straus, E., Tetroe, J., & Graham, I. (2009). Defining knowledge translation. *Canadian Medical Association Journal*, *181*(3–4), 165–168.

Taylor, R. (2020). *The intentional relationship; occupational therapy and use of self.* F.A. Davis.

Taylor, R. R., Lee, S. W., Kielhofner, G., & Ketkar, M. (2009). Therapeutic use of self: a nationwide survey of practitioners' attitudes and experiences. *American Journal of Occupational Therapy*, *63*(2), 198–207.

Walder, K., Bissett, M., Molineux, M., & Whiteford, G. (2022). Understanding professional identity in occupational therapy: a scoping review. *Scandinavian Journal of Occupational Therapy*, *3*, 175–197.

CHAPTER 4

Using the Expertise of Others: Many Hands Make Light Work

Accessing Knowledge from Others to Inform Professional Decisions

Elizabeth Martin

Senior Lecturer, School of Occupational Therapy, Te Pūkenga|Otago Polytechnic, New Zealand

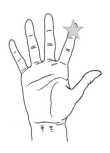

INTRODUCTION

In the Five Finger Framework (FFF), the index finger represents the expertise of others and the influence this can have on decisions made within professional reasoning processes. The expertise of others, added to what we already know, can facilitate the development of knowledge and skills, and provide reassurance. Tapping into expert knowledge is a natural way of learning and reflects social learning theory, as developed by Albert Bandura and now known as social cognitive theory (Weiten, 2017). A component of this theory is observational learning, where Bandura described four stages necessary for learning to take place: attention, retention, reproduction, and motivation. In this theory, learning occurs through the social elements of listening, observing, conversing, and questioning of others as people participate in the world and interact with others (Rolls et al., 2016). Bandura suggested behavior is shaped by the people we are exposed to, thus when we are exposed to and observe the expertise of others, we can learn from them. It is widely acknowledged that observing role models is an effective way to learn in the health field; learners internalize what they see and hear so they can reproduce the behavior (Horsburgh & Ippolito, 2018; Naidoo & Van Wyk, 2016).

Accessing the expertise of others can be facilitated directly and indirectly. Direct access can be through supervision and access to experienced colleagues and peers who can be questioned and assist with decision making (Jeffery et al., 2021). This form of learning can be intentional, such as through direct questioning of others, or fortuitous, such as some of the effects of observing and mentoring. The way others operate influences our understanding of how things are done; thus, those with expertise can significantly influence the professional reasoning and decision making of others. Indirect access can be through online materials and platforms, and conferences that enable access to known international experts.

Within the FFF, the index finger is a prompt to encourage questioning of experts, asking "who can help me with this decision?" and "how best can I access their expertise?," both of which are explored in this chapter.

Setting the Scene

I am a recently graduated physiotherapist. My first position is on the orthopedic ward of a local hospital where I work closely with clinicians from several disciplines, including occupational therapy, medicine, nursing, and social work. I feel fortunate that the clinical nurse manager on the ward fosters an environment that encourages questioning and supports the sharing of knowledge between the disciplines, which has been found to be hugely helpful

for novice practitioners such as myself (Jeffery et al., 2021). Our clients cover a variety of ages and conditions, with their length of stay on the unit ranging from overnight to several weeks. I have learned a little about the FFF during my physiotherapy training and can see significant benefits of using it within my current setting. I plan to introduce the framework to the multidisciplinary team on the unit using one of my clients, Julie, to demonstrate how together we can use it to enhance our practice.

WHO IS THE CLIENT?

Julie is 53 years old and has lived with her female partner, Susan, for the past nine years. She was admitted to the orthopedic ward with multiple fractures in her right leg and left wrist following a road traffic accident. She was traveling home from her job as a high school teacher on her motorcycle when hit by a car. She has had external fixation surgery to her lower right leg, and a metal rod inserted in her femur. Her left wrist is in a cast.

When I received Julie's referral, I was looking forward to helping her recover from severe injuries and major surgery; however, I was also nervous. I had read articles and textbooks about severe fractures and the different potential treatment plans involved (literature and research finger), but my only experience of working with clients who had external fixators fitted was as a student on fieldwork placement. I was aware that this time, *I* would be the physiotherapist working with Julie, rather than my placement supervisors as in the past. There would be several decisions I would need to make; this would really test my professional reasoning. I felt sure I would need the knowledge and expertise of others to ensure the best outcome for Julie.

ACCESSING EXPERTISE WITHIN THE WORK SETTING

I first met Julie as she lay on her hospital bed in the orthopedic ward the day after her surgery. She was visibly upset at what had happened to her, explaining that she had never been in hospital before and had no idea how she was going to cope with the coming days, weeks, and months. After talking with Julie and outlining what the beginning stages of her rehabilitation would involve, she broke down into tears and asked me to leave. I was at a loss at what to do next, and sought advice from Heather, our clinical nurse manager. Heather had been responsible for the overall running of the unit for the past 12 years and was vastly experienced. She was particularly respected for the relationships she was able to quickly build with patients, something I had witnessed and admired.

Heather asked if I would like to accompany her as she met with Julie so that I could observe and learn from her practice, a vital stage of social learning theory (Horsburgh & Ippolito, 2018). I jumped at this opportunity and watched as Heather used her skills to put Julie at ease, demonstrating the person-centered practice central to the client's insight finger.

The first thing I noticed was how Heather took the time to clear some of the hospital equipment that had built up on the chair next to Julie's bed and how she positioned herself there. This enabled Heather to be at the same level as Julie, rather than standing over her as I had done. Heather informed me later that she had done this to let Julie know that she was happy to spend time talking with her, rather than giving the impression she was so busy she would be off to attend to another task soon. In this way, I felt Julie valued the session and was more inclined to share how she was feeling at her own pace. I also observed the tone of voice Heather used. Even though Julie began crying again and was clearly agitated, Heather responded with a calm tone which did not change throughout the whole interaction. I noticed Julie visibly relaxing as Heather interacted with her to gain her trust. Such role modeling of practice skills has been found to influence novices such as myself (Jeffery et al., 2021; Vinales, 2015). Although Heather was from an alternative discipline, her skills were fully transferable and something I wanted to integrate into my practice. At my next meeting with Julie, I remembered some of the strategies Heather had used; I reproduced these myself, making our interactions much more positive. Through observing Heather's practice and then trying this myself, I was able to support Julie as she slowly moved from a supine position to sitting on the edge of the bed.

I knew the next stage was for Julie to move to an upright position, and then begin to mobilize around the ward. I was concerned about how to assist Julie to mobilize most effectively, particularly the best mobility aid to use. I felt confident when educating clients on how to use a walking frame or crutches when they had fractures in one of their lower limbs. However, the fact that Julie not only had multiple leg fractures but also a fractured wrist meant that her situation was different from any I had encountered before. I was concerned that Julie was not able to take weight through her left wrist and so the equipment I had used before, such as crutches or a two-wheel/two stopper frame, would not be appropriate. I thought someone with expertise in mobilizing clients with more complex needs would be the best person to help.

There are several physiotherapists who work in different areas of the hospital, one of whom, Debbie, is my assigned mentor and supervisor. She was currently based on the rehabilitation unit but has worked in all areas of the hospital at various times, meaning she is familiar with the practice environment (context finger). Over our lunch break, I made a point of explaining Julie's situation to Debbie and asked her advice regarding the best course of action. Debbie suggested I initially try a forearm support frame so that Julie could weight bear through her forearms. Together, Debbie and I located a suitable frame and I felt confident this would be the best course of action to take with Julie. I felt grateful for and supported by the mentorship model of my workplace – accessing others to help with my professional reasoning enabled safer and more appropriate decisions on my part.

The next time I went to see Julie, I brought the frame with me. However, as soon as she saw it, she became visibly tense and informed me she was not ready to try it. This was difficult for me as I knew how important it was for her to be mobilizing as quickly as possible. Fortunately, Jacky, an experienced occupational therapist based on the ward, saw what was happening and came over. She had spent some time with Julie, getting to know her personality and her home situation (linking to client finger). Jacky reminded me how important it can be to involve a client's family in their therapy and relayed how much Julie relied on her partner, Susan, for emotional support. Jacky indicated that Susan would play a vital part in Julie's rehabilitation and suggested I ask if she could be present the next time Julie attempted to mobilize. Susan was delighted to be able to help and agreed to join us. I observed how Jacky involved Susan in the session, giving her time to reassure Julie so that she was more confident and relaxed when mobilizing for the first time. The next time I assisted Julie to mobilize, I ensured Susan was available to be there for support. This also emphasized for me just how much helpful knowledge is held within the family and immediate social group of the client – expertise is not just the domain of professionals!

As a novice, having colleagues available for help as I worked out what I should be doing to best help Julie enhanced my own practice and clinical safety (Jeffery et al., 2021) and enabled me to make sense of the knowledge I had gained in my studies and through my reading (literature finger) (Li et al., 2009).

SUPERVISION

I experienced a lot of learning in a short space of time with Julie, so I took her case to my next supervision session. As a newly graduated practitioner, I sometimes have difficulty with my professional reasoning, a situation common for novices (Naidoo & Van Wyk, 2016), and so appreciated the opportunity to check in with Debbie. Talking to my supervisor highlighted how I had been applying the FFF to my practice. Debbie was not aware of this framework and was impressed with the way I had used it to inform my decision making. She suggested I introduce the framework to the physiotherapy team at one of our fortnightly professional development meetings. I was a little apprehensive, but Debbie assured me the whole team could benefit from my sharing of knowledge and so I looked forward to presenting at an in-service session. As I was talking to Debbie, it struck me that our supervision session was in fact another aspect of the expertise of others finger in action!

Clinical supervision has been found to be effective in enhancing professional development and client care for allied health professionals (Gardner et al., 2018). I am grateful for supervision within a structured framework at a set time each week that is guided by a supervision agreement as this is reported to result in supervision being most effective (Saxby et al., 2015). I have opportunities to reflect on my practice and discuss a range of issues. In this way, I can talk through my professional reasoning decisions and gain a lot from Debbie's experience and input.

COLLABORATIVE DECISION MAKING

I knew that Julie would not spend much time on the ward, as there was always pressure on beds and early discharge was encouraged (context finger). We would need to decide if she could go home soon or if her situation warranted transfer to the longer-term rehabilitation ward. I felt anxious about this decision, as I had no idea really whether she could manage at home or not. However, we had a weekly case conference meeting, and it is here that interdisciplinary team decisions are made collaboratively. "The intent of interprofessional collaboration is that clinicians work deliberatively together with the patient and family to provide optimal healthcare" (Costanzo et al., 2019, p. 185). To honor this process, wherever possible the patient is included in this meeting.

Here information is shared about the decision to be made, the benefits and risks of options and what best practice guidelines indicate. The patient's values and preferences are considered along with the professional perspective of the interdisciplinary team members. The decision is intentionally deliberated by the group who are mutually informed of both the decision and the best evidence, able to integrate patient values and knowledge and

come to a mutually agreed plan (Costanzo et al., 2019). This meeting clearly demonstrated the expertise we all hold as professionals, and the specialism that sits with each discipline. Importantly, it illustrated how crucial it is to integrate this with the expertise held by the client and family, so that plans are possible in the client's context (environment finger).

KNOWLEDGE TRANSLATION

Knowledge translation describes the "movement" of knowledge from its creation to a point of direct influence on clinical practice (Kitson & Harvey, 2016). The aim of knowledge translation is to enhance both the "use and usefulness of research" (Wensing & Grol, 2019, p. 1). While working with Julie, I had in the back of my mind that I was unaware of the latest best practice research when working with a client with external fixators. I knew the importance of using literature, but I just seemed so busy that taking time to search for it, let alone read it, felt overwhelming.

Debbie reminded me of our knowledge translator, Lucas. For one day a week, Lucas works alongside our hospital librarian with the aim of locating current research relevant to our practice areas (lit/research finger). This knowledge can then be disseminated and integrated into intervention processes, reflecting how knowledge translation strategies can impact the actions of clinicians by increasing the link between evidence and practice (Barwick et al., 2009).

I shared with Lucas how I wanted to find the latest literature regarding best practice for a client with external fixators. Lucas was able to identify and share research related to this topic which I was then able to integrate into my treatment plan. This helped me to feel confident that the decisions I made with Julie were based on reliable evidence. It did still take some time and effort on my part, and so I wrote up my summary of best current evidence to share with my colleagues, in the hope that it may help them in the future. My manager was impressed with this, added it to our evidence folder and at the next staff meeting thanked me for the work.

I had been talking about the FFF with my peers, and here was an opportunity to talk about how research evidence (literature finger) can be incorporated into workplace resources and systems (environment finger) and enables us to share our specialties (expertise of others finger). The ensuing conversation was motivating for everyone in the meeting, and we decided as a group that we would all contribute to the folder.

COMMUNITIES OF PRACTICE

Barwick et al. (2009) stated that "knowledge translation needs to be situated within the context in which it will be used and developed" (p. 27) which was evident in my involvement in a community of practice (CoP) focused on orthopedic care. Within the health sector, CoPs are intended to facilitate knowledge exchange across boundaries to generate a body of knowledge accessible by members. They are intended to promote learning and thus improve practice (Ranmuthugala et al., 2011). The way CoPs are organized and operated varies significantly, but they generally consist of an informal learning organization or network (Li et al., 2009). This is the case for the CoP of which I am a member. I joined the CoP after being invited by my final student placement supervisor. The group consists of health professionals who are passionate about the rehabilitation of individuals requiring therapy for an orthopedic issue. I see this as a wonderful way to learn from

the expertise of others and have also invited others on the ward to join.

A group of us, recognizing we have shared knowledge and an identity within the practice community (Ranmuthugala et al., 2011; Rolls et al., 2016), meet using video call at an agreed time each month. Virtual communities such as this include individuals who use an online platform to share experiences and professional expertise (Shaw et al., 2022). During these meetings, we communicate information and insights, advise each other, solve problems, and consider common issues (Wenger et al., 2002). CoPs such as this provide a safe environment and contribute to improved rates of implementation of evidence-based practice (McLoughlin et al., 2017). Also, the social nature of our live discussions means there is a sense of community between all those who attend (Shaw et al., 2022). Moreover, the fact that we meet online means that geographical location is not a barrier (Struminger et al., 2017), as our members are located all over the country.

As a new graduate, I have found this group to be invaluable; I have learnt from practitioners from a variety of disciplines, with years of experience between them. It has been immensely beneficial to hear the perspectives of other physiotherapists, but also those of other health disciplines who are part of the CoP. Within this "social structure. . . based on mutual respect, trust, and information sharing" (Kothari et al., 2015, p. 2), I shared some details regarding Julie's condition and treatment. Through discussion with members in the group, I was able to make sense of the articles and textbooks I had read related to serious fractures (literature finger) and apply this to the context of my practice with Julie (Li et al., 2009). Through tapping into the knowledge of the group members, I expanded my own knowledge and appreciated how we were able to adjust the agenda of our meetings to suit my needs (Barwick et al., 2009).

The internet, a part of everyday life for health professionals, is useful for networking and sharing knowledge (Rolls et al., 2016) and extending professionalism (Laliberte et al., 2016; McLoughlin et al., 2017). Research into often used social media platforms in professional work has shown that they can enhance professional development, cultivate collegiality, and help circulate research and public health information (Laliberte et al., 2016; Ward et al., 2018).

I have felt many of these benefits through my participation in a social media group consisting of physiotherapists practicing in my local area. Asynchronous communication enabled by social media accessible on a variety of devices enables us to post whenever we get a moment, and to check regularly to see what the latest thinking regarding physiotherapy practice is (McLoughlin et al., 2017). Those who contribute cover a broad range of experience and practice areas, and so it is a fantastic way to learn from others from the same profession. For example, during my lunchbreak, I used my phone to add a post asking for the thoughts of others regarding their experiences working with clients with multiple lower limb fractures. That evening, and throughout the next day, other physiotherapists added their thoughts and suggested readings which may be beneficial (literature finger). I was then able to apply this knowledge to my own clinical context. The literature also reports that virtual communities of practice are becoming more focused on sharing and promoting evidence-based practice due to members drawing on expertise from clinical experience, research, clients, and the local context (McLoughlin et al., 2017).

I really benefitted from the "explicit and experiential knowledge" (McLoughlin et al., 2017, p. 139) that was shared. Using the expertise of physiotherapists outside the hospital setting gave me more confidence with my decision making when working with Julie, knowing that it was based on current best practice within my discipline (Rolls et al., 2016).

ONLINE ACCESS TO EXPERTISE OF OTHERS

I was also able to access the expertise of others through attendance at an online physiotherapy conference. I was particularly encouraged to attend because one of the keynote speakers was a physiotherapist based in a region close to where I live. This meant her presentation was during my normal work hours, so I did not have to navigate an unreasonable time during the early hours of the morning, and I felt more connected as her name was familiar to me. Both factors have been found to generate increased attendance at online conferences (Hoffman et al., 2021). One of the most beneficial features of the conference was the ability to ask questions in the chat, a practice that has been shown to encourage attendee participation (Roos et al., 2020). I was able to raise the topic of the impact of external fixators on rehabilitation and hear the opinions of a very well-respected member of our profession. As a novice practitioner, the decisions I made with Julie were enhanced by the views of the speaker.

In addition, I have been able to listen to the views of a renowned American physiotherapist, via the Technology, Entertainment and Design Talks (TED Talks); within this online platform, ideas and research are presented by a variety of speakers (MacKrill et al., 2021). A particular professor I am aware of who is recognized as a top expert in his field frequently speaks on the topic of supporting individuals through the initial stages of recovery after severe injury.

He speaks with passion and energy in an entertaining way, a situation common with TED Talks (Masson, 2014). Geographical and financial constraints mean personally attending one of his keynote conference addresses would be impossible, but his TED Talks are freely available at any time. He has also featured on a physiotherapy-focused podcast I regularly listen to. Through these two mediums, I have listened to and learned from the expertise of this professor and use this knowledge to inform my own practice.

PEER LEARNING

In contrast to learning from established, internationally renowned physiotherapists, I was also able to access the expertise of other new graduate physiotherapists with whom I had completed my training. The constructivist approach to peer learning theory inherent in Vygotsky's sociocultural theory stresses the value of learning through collaborative dialogs (Weiten, 2017). Although Vygotsky's research focused on children, his theory can also be applied to adults (Shah & Rashidas, 2017) as demonstrated by the communication with my former classmates. I have been able to share my concerns and learn through conversations over Facetime, Facebook messenger, text messages, and phone calls. Although they would not consider themselves "experts" in that they had only recently graduated, they nevertheless had experiences and understanding that were of benefit to me. Additionally, we were all "in the same boat" in terms of negotiating the new world of practising as a registered physiotherapist. Applying this peer learning strategy, combined with my increasing experience in the field, has increased the range of clinical practice skills I am able to draw on, and thus improved my clinical decision making (Naidoo & Van Wyk, 2016).

SHARING THE BENEFITS OF THE FIVE FINGER FRAMEWORK AT IN-SERVICE SESSIONS

I was able to present on the benefits of the FFF at our in-service session, which was very well received by my colleagues. I suggested the following ideas related to practitioners including students, service managers, supervisors, and educators (Figure 4.1).

Role	Key Points
Practitioner/ student	• Recognize the benefits of accessing the expertise of others from other disciplines. • Participate in relevant CoPs. • Access online expertise, e.g., TED Talks, podcasts. • Research possibilities to attend conferences, both in person and virtually. • Keep up to date with current research and transfer knowledge into practice. • Be open to learning from the expertise of others in all its different forms. • Take note of the practice of others around you, and reflect on the learning involved. • Locate relevant literature, discuss with supervisor, and put directly into practice (knowledge translation).

Role	Key Points
Manager	• Allow opportunities for within- and cross-discipline liaison to facilitate learning from the expertise of others, e.g., provide professional development time. • Employ knowledge translators within the setting or establish knowledge translation processes. • Provide mentors for new graduate practitioners. • Enable collaborative decision making. • Embed the Five Finger Framework in the service as a way of promoting broad professional reasoning and a shared language between all staff.
Supervisor	• Be open to different forms of supervision dependent on the needs and learning style of students. • Provide opportunities for students to ask questions. • Provide opportunities for students to observe practice and then put what they have learned into their interactions with clients. • Use the Five Finger Framework to structure some supervision sessions.
Educator	• Highlight to students the variety of expertise available to them. • Role play situations of learning from colleagues through observation – feedback on learning identified. • Students to identify conditions/situations within case studies and research any relevant online material, e.g., TED Talks, podcasts, online conferences. • Educate regarding the ways in which supervision can be used to assist with clinical reasoning.

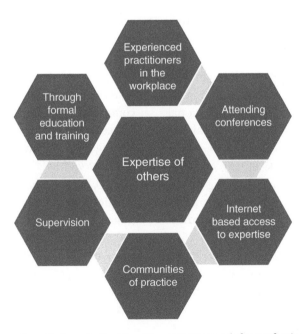

FIGURE 4.1   The expertise of others in the Five Finger Framework for professional reasoning.

This chapter has highlighted the value of using the expertise of others to inform and strengthen our professional reasoning. Importantly, the breadth of opportunities and resources we have at our fingertips to access this expertise is illustrated. On the FFF, the next (middle) finger represents the person or client and explores both how useful and essential it is to maintain a collaborative focus between practitioner and client in professional reasoning processes. This is illustrated in the next chapter.

REFERENCES

Barwick, M. A., Peters, J., & Boydell, K. (2009). Getting to uptake: do communities of practice support the implementation of evidence-based practice? *Journal of the Canadian Academy of Child and Adolescent Psychiatry*, 18(1), 16–29.

Costanzo, C., Doll, J., & Jensen, G. M. (2019). Shared decision making in practice. In J. Higgs, G. M. Jensen, S. Loftus, & N. Christensen (Eds.), *Clinical reasoning in the health professions* (pp. 181–190). Elsevier.

Gardner, M. J., McKinstry, C., & Perrin, B. (2018). Effectiveness of allied health clinical supervision. A cross-sectional survey of supervisees. *Journal of Allied Health*, 47(2), 126–132.

Hoffman, D. L., Paek, S., Ho, C. P., & Kimura, B. Y. (2021). Online-only international conferences: strategies for maintaining community. *TechTrends*, 65(4), 418–420.

Horsburgh, J., & Ippolito, K. (2018). A skill to be worked at: using social learning theory to explore the process of learning from role models in clinical settings. *BMC Medical Education*, 18(1), article number 156

Jeffery, H., Robertson, L., & Reay, K. L. (2021). Sources of evidence for professional decision-making in novice occupational therapy practitioners: clinicians' perspectives. *British Journal of Occupational Therapy*, 84(6), 346–354.

Kitson, A. L. &., & Harvey, G. (2016). Methods to succeed in effective knowledge translation in clinical practice. *Journal of Nursing Scholarship*, 48(3), 294–302.

Kothari, A., Boyko, J. A., Conklin, J., Stolee, P., & Sibbald, S. L. (2015). Communities of practice for supporting health systems change: a missed opportunity. *Health Research Policy and Systems*, 13(1), 33.

Laliberté, M., Beaulieu-Poulin, C., Campeau Larrivée, A., Charbonneau, M., Samson, É., & Ehrmann Feldman, D. (2016). Current uses (and potential misuses) of Facebook: an online survey in physiotherapy. *Physiotherapy Canada*, 68(1), 5–12.

Li, L. C., Grimshaw, J. M., Nielsen, C., Judd, M., Coyte, P. C., & Graham, I. D. (2009). Evolution of Wenger's concept of community of practice. *Implementation Science*, 4(1), 11.

MacKrill, K., Silvester, C., Pennebaker, J. W., & Petrie, K. J. (2021). What makes an idea worth spreading? Language markers of popularity in TED talks by academics and other speakers. *Journal of the Association for Information Science and Technology*, 72(8), 1028–1038.

Masson, M. (2014). Benefits of TED talks. *Canadian Family Physician*, 60(12), 1080.

McLoughlin, C., Patel, K. D., O'Callaghan, T., & Reeves, S. (2017). The use of virtual communities of practice to improve interprofessional collaboration and education: findings from an integrated review. *Journal of Interprofessional Care*, 32(2), 136–142.

Naidoo, D., & Van Wyk, J. (2016). Fieldwork practice for learning: lessons from occupational therapy students and their supervisors. *African Journal of Health Professions Education*, 8(1), 37–40.

Ranmuthugala, G., Plumb, J. J., Cunningham, F. C., Georgiou, A., Westbrook, J. I., & Braithwaite, J. (2011). How and why are communities of practice established in the healthcare sector? A systematic review of the literature. *BMC Health Services Research, 11*, 273.

Rolls, K., Hansen, M., Jackson, D., & Elliott, D. (2016). How health care professionals use social media to create virtual communities: an integrative review. *Journal of Medical Internet Research, 18*(6), e166.

Roos, G., Oláh, J., Ingle, R., Kobayashi, M., & Feldt, M. (2020). Online conferences – towards a new (virtual) reality. *Computational and Theoretical Chemistry, 1189*, 112975.

Saxby, C., Wilson, J., & Newcombe, P. (2015). Can clinical supervision sustain our workforce in the current healthcare landscape? Findings from a Queensland study of allied health professionals. *Australian Health Review, 39*(4), 476–482.

Shah, T., & Rashid, S. (2017). Applying Vygotsky to adult learning. *Journal of Social Sciences, 8*, 1–13.

Shaw, L., Jazayeri, D., Kiegaldie, D., & Morris, M. E. (2022). Implementation of virtual communities of practice in healthcare to improve capability and capacity: a 10-year scoping review. *International Journal of Environmental Research and Public Health, 19*(13), 7994.

Struminger, B., Arora, S., Zalud-Cerrato, S., Lowrance, D., & Ellerbrock, T. (2017). Building virtual communities of practice for health. *Lancet, 390*(10095), 632–634.

Vinales, J. J. (2015). The mentor as a role model and the importance of belongingness. *British Journal of Nursing, 24*(10), 532–535.

Ward, A., Eng, C., McCue, V., Stewart, R., Strain, K., McCormack, B., Dukhu, S., Thomas, J., & Bulley, C. (2018). What matters versus what's the matter – exploring perceptions of person-centred practice in nursing and physiotherapy social media communities: a qualitative study. *International Practice Development Journal, 8*(2), 3.

Weiten, W. (2017). *Psychology: Themes and variations* (10th ed.). Cengage Learning.

Wenger, E., McDermott, R., & Snyder, W. M. (2002). *Cultivating communities of practice.* Harvard Business School Press.

Wensing, M., & Grol, R. (2019). Knowledge translation in health: how implementation science could contribute more. *BMC Medicine, 17*(1), 88.

CHAPTER 5

Walking Hand in Hand: Collaborative Practice

Eliciting and Incorporating Client Perspectives

Helen Jeffery

Principal Lecturer, School of Occupational Therapy, Te Pūkenga|Otago Polytechnic, New Zealand

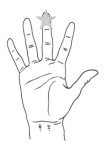

INTRODUCTION

An integral element of the Five Finger Framework (FFF) is forming a collaborative relationship with the person or people receiving the health intervention. This includes ascertaining their perspective and expertise and integrating this into professional reasoning processes. The person(s) (or client[s]) is represented on the FFF by the middle and tallest finger, situated centrally, with the intention that they remain central to all decisions made. The term "person" is used interchangeably with "client" throughout this chapter and refers to the person, people, group, or community accessing the service. Who is brought to the therapy process and how they work together with the therapist profoundly influence the decisions made by the therapist on a day-to-day basis.

The client perspective is integral to evidence-based practice, illustrated by Sackett et al.'s (2000) definition: ". . .the integration of best available evidence, clinical expertise and patient preferences and values." Person-centered practice arises from a humanistic perspective and has its roots in the work of Carl Rogers (1986) who proposed that ". . . the individual has within himself or herself vast resources for self-understanding, for altering his or her self-concept, attitudes, and self-directed behaviour – and that these resources can be tapped...." (pp. 115–117). Rogers was instrumental in developing an approach where therapists work from a paradigm of understanding the person as in need of an empathetic relationship that facilitates a feeling of being understood and valued. In such a relationship, the person can move toward growth and development. Principles of person-centered practice form the basis for collaboration between the person and practitioner or service.

This chapter explores ways in which practitioners can maintain a view where the person is central to intervention through appreciating their position and perspective, utilizing the expertise they bring, and being culturally safe in their practice. This is evident in the collaborative relationship between practitioner and client and in interventions the practitioner selects to empower people they work with. Additionally, the client is involved in background processes that enable this way of working (such as feedback-informed processes), and client education to inform and enhance collaboration in the practice decisions made.

Although straightforward to understand, person-centered practice can be difficult to integrate into a practitioner's way of thinking and working. It is sometimes considered a threshold concept (Meyer & Land, 2003) which is a concept that, once grasped, is transformational in the way an element of professional practice is viewed. The "threshold" many practitioners need to cross for this concept is from a view that the practitioner does "to" or "for" the person using their expertise to a view that they are doing "with" the person. So, the essence of person-centered practice is in the practitioner and client forming a relationship where they can work together.

Setting the Scene

I am a speech and language therapist with four years' experience and have recently started a new job in a small inner-city practice. We primarily work with people who have experienced a stroke and have significant communication and perceptual issues as a result. Most of our clients are older people and recently discharged from the inpatient neurological rehabilitation unit; many are in residential care. This work is funded through the hospital system, and we have considerable autonomy over the service we provide. We occasionally work with younger clients through contracts to a large health insurance company. Marty, a 37-year-old manager of a large inner-city business, was my first such client. I am familiar with the FFF as a framework for assisting my professional reasoning and use this to help me through decisions as they emerge.

WHO IS THE CLIENT?

On receiving the referral for Marty, I started to think about how different it would be working with a younger person in a different life stage. He had sustained trauma to his neck in a car accident which led to a cerebral vascular accident (CVA) with damage to the Broca's area. His associated Broca's aphasia was the primary communication issue; whilst able to string some sentences together, he had considerable difficulty word finding. He also had some right-sided weakness affecting his overall function and, importantly for my work, moderate dysarthria resulting in slurred speech.

Although I had little information to go on at this stage, I needed an intervention plan for approval by my manager. I mapped out and presented my planned assessment process and intervention strategies and was distressed to discover it was unrealistic because of the timeframe. I had planned more than the allocated one session a week, for a six-week period. Whilst more than six sessions might be applied for, there was no guarantee it would be approved. Thinking about the influence of the environment (context finger) in professional reasoning, I realized I had not appreciated the direct influence this factor should have had on my planning. The insurer was also my client, so I needed to provide the service as contracted with them. This created an uncomfortable dissonance for me – I appreciated the need for efficient and cost-effective service and felt loyalty to the organization paying the bills. However, I equally felt a strong allegiance to Marty who was struggling. I knew I had knowledge and skills that would be helpful for his recovery. I needed to be able to tease out what the issues were and ensure that despite demands on my time and resources, I could maintain a position where Marty remained front of mind in my decision making and where I could make best use of my knowledge and skills (the self – thumb).

Marty arrived for his initial assessment appointment accompanied by his wife, his mother, and an uncle, all of whom insisted on being involved during the session. They had no qualms about providing me with information regarding the impact of his stroke on the family and of what they would do for Marty to help them get through this crisis. Once I settled into understanding the collectivist nature of their Asian ethnicity (Marty's parents were first-generation immigrants to my culturally Eurocentric homeland), I began to appreciate the influence of my individualist approach to the therapy I usually provided. I was reminded that although the client may be the person who has been referred to the service, there are times where this view is muddied.

Many Indigenous cultures consider that the health challenge pertains to the family and expect assessment and intervention to be conducted with family members present as well as the individual with the need. Touching base with family can enhance understanding of presenting issues. Both context and history are available to augment documented information within the health system and what the clients themselves have to say. Understanding the family's collective view of illness and approach to coping is important, although the information needs to be expertly juggled. Individuals might disclose more when they have family members present, or less if they are not willing for family to be fully aware of what is going on for them. The complexity of family culture and relationships needs to be considered when offering appointments with extended family. Ethical considerations emerge in terms of privacy, including what to document, who can access that information, client autonomy, and weighing up their wishes alongside family information, and managing information the person shares that is helpful for professional reasoning but not directly required for the assessment or intervention.

Ensuring I developed and maintained a person-centered approach to my work with Marty and his family whilst manipulating multiple sources of potentially helpful information was going to be challenging. Equally challenging would be considering this family's beliefs and values regarding health and recovery within the Eurocentric influence of the system and culture I was embedded in.

Marty was 37 years old, he had a wife, two children, a mortgage, and a career. Whilst his aphasia and associated communication issues presented like other people I was working with, the impact on his life was dramatically different because of his life stage. Again, the nuanced understanding of who my client was shifted. I had worked in a previous job with children experiencing developmental communication issues – my approach with them had been quite different from the older and retired population in my current role. This was of course in part due to the nature of the presenting problems, but also their life stage and the complicating factor of having parents, caregivers, and schoolteachers to include in the "who is the client" conundrum. Marty was my first experience working with someone who had the pressure of returning to work, providing for family, and meeting financial demands.

One thing I had in my favor was my experience with people recovering from a stroke which has helped me develop specialized knowledge of treating the associated speech and communication disorders. This enabled me to ask pertinent questions and to quickly build a picture of what he was experiencing. My ability to probe for specific issues helped me feel empathy for Marty and helped with relationship building – he and his family members seemed to relax and to show signs of trust once they knew how informed I was.

Reflecting on this takes me back to my early days working in neurorehabilitation and primarily with people who had experienced a stroke. Those first months were intense and the information I needed to handle felt overwhelming. The needs that people presented with were diverse and layered with complexity. Although there were similarities in some of the communication challenges and these matched the textbook information, there remained vast diversity between individual people. In terms of the FFF, I found myself focusing on the research and literature finger quite often as I worked out the best research evidence-based practice. Each assessment, intervention decision, and plan took an inordinate amount of

time and cognitive energy for me. How to handle all the information and form an understanding of what was going on for the person and my place in assisting in their recovery seemed out of reach. I was very reliant on my colleagues and supervisor for assistance (expertise of others finger). I felt fortunate that I had learned how to use supervision effectively.

My supervisor encouraged me to analyze the health condition using literature, and to look for patterns in what I was seeing. This formal health condition analysis helped me understand the onset of the condition/s, signs and symptoms, etiology, prognosis, etc. Using a template to guide this and having developed a habit of using this when starting in a new practice area or when receiving a referral for someone who has a diagnosis unfamiliar to me helps me gain a quick appreciation of what to observe and enquire about when meeting the person. Gradually, I came to understand CVA and, importantly, likely issues related to speech, communication, and swallowing. Patterns emerged in what I was experiencing with the clients, I made links, I could anticipate specific issues and develop effective interventions.

This knowledge of general presenting issues, usual course of the condition, and likely prognosis and intervention pathway has become crucial in helping me appreciate the client's perspective, being able to assess and communicate with people in an informed way and thus to plan appropriate assessment and intervention strategies. To develop my understanding of this health condition, I have also spent time with or listening to individuals with lived experience of CVA which has helped gain insight into their perspective – many of the people I work with are in residential facilities and I can be with them in their everyday environment. I also attend a support group as a volunteer and have met with advocacy groups. Additionally, internet resources, conferences where service users present, and publications written by people with lived experience have been enlightening for me. The Database of Individual Patients' Experiences' (DIPEx Charity, 2023) is a particularly useful website that draws together information about conditions and clients' experiences, and facilitates working relationships between clients and researchers.

I know that ways to enable clients to lend a helping hand in our understanding of their experience are developing rapidly as we move from a prescriptive stance to partnership-based relationships. I have also noticed that employing client advocates and including client voices in service development and planning are also advancing the movement toward person- or family-centered services.

RELATIONSHIP FIRST

An honest, genuine, and respectful relationship is central to person-centered practice. Research from psychotherapy literature has shown that it is the relationship between person and therapist that has most effect in counseling and psychotherapy, rather than the therapy approach used (Baldwin et al., 2007). The extent to which this is the case depends on the profession and the nature of the service being provided. However, all health interventions will be positively affected by the development of an effective therapeutic relationship.

Using a model or framework to help with learning to form and maintain professional relationships is helpful to many, particularly novice practitioners. The Intentional Relationship Model (Taylor, 2020) is an example, where interpersonal characteristics of the person are explored (such as their level of trust or need for control), alongside interpersonal events that commonly arise

in client–practitioner interactions (e.g., intimate self-disclosure, boundary testing). Additionally, ways to navigate these events are explored, and options regarding specific modes of relating to a client (advocating, collaborating, empathizing, encouraging, instructing, and problem solving) are outlined.

Forming a relationship with Marty felt like a challenge when I started working with him as this was my first experience of working with someone immersed in a traditional family structure and involved in a wider community that operated in a way that was quite different from my cultural "norm." This experience prompted me to direct my attention to the thumb (use of self) and reflect on my own beliefs, values, and culture, in particular the individualist lens I saw the world through, so that I could better appreciate the differences between our way of being in society that might influence our relationship.

The foundation for collaboration is mutual respect and shared responsibility for the therapy process. I took myself to the research and literature finger and searched for literature related to stroke and speech and language therapy. This was clarifying for me, particularly in understanding some of the challenges in using client narratives when working with people with communication issues, and ways in which we can develop partnership in our work (Forsgren et al., 2022). Much of the success in building an effective relationship is down to communication skills. I had learned some specific communication strategies through learning about Motivational Interviewing (MI) (Miller & Rollnick, 2012) but I had never been in a situation where my relationship so clearly needed to be with the extended family rather than the individual. I had always ensured I communicated with family members whenever appropriate, but this experience illustrated just how superficial my relationships with families of clients had been in the past. They were just that – the families of clients, rather than the family being the client. Perhaps refreshing my knowledge of MI and using those strategies with Marty and his family would be helpful.

I understood that the overall ethos and specific strategies of MI have been guided by person-centeredness. The "Spirit of Motivational Interviewing" incorporates collaboration between practitioner and person, with the practitioner evoking motivation for change through facilitating the person's own awareness of reasons to change and honoring their autonomy (Miller & Rollnick, 2012). When learning to use the strategies, I had been surprised at the impact on my capacity for listening with empathy and the focus I developed on empowering the person and understanding their motivations. Whilst MI was developed specifically for eliciting health behavioral change, I think that the communication style is appropriate for all health providers in most settings. I learned therapeutic communication skills in my undergraduate education, but this additional knowledge in MI equipped me with skills to enact a person-centered approach in my work. Importantly, the strategies are useful in guiding the establishment of a relationship that places the person at the center without crossing the boundary into personal relationship.

Appreciating what is appropriate to share with clients is always complex. I could see this would be difficult for me with Marty's family as they got to know and accept me into their team. Hopefully, my intentional use of MI strategies would help me navigate the boundary between personal and professional relationships, and ensure the focus remained on the speech and language therapy I could offer.

COLLABORATION

Shared decision making is fundamental to a working partnership. It is important to develop a mutual understanding of the extent to which the client wishes to engage in the decision-making process regarding intervention. This varies depending in part on the nature of the issue. For example, in the acute phase the person may prefer to hand responsibility for decisions over to the practitioner but in the rehabilitation phase they may wish to have much more input, depending on the life stage the person is in and if the service is short term (recovery) or long term (e.g., developmental or palliative), and cultural factors, e.g., expectation that the professional will provide expert instruction and set the goals for the intervention. Equally, the beliefs the person holds regarding their health, wellbeing, and recovery will play a part in how engaged they are in sharing decisions (Vahdat et al., 2014).

One way in which I worked toward collaboration was through conversation with Marty where I tried to hear his story, to get a feel for his past and current situation and where he saw himself going and how he thought he would get there. This narrative approach to reasoning is useful when forming collaborative relationships – Marty's stories helped me work out how to weave my therapy in so that his envisaged future became a part of our goals, that he felt hope, and so that I had a gradually developing sophisticated picture of the story Marty is now living out (Hamilton, 2018; Mattingly & Flemming, 2019). "Listening" in this instance involved noticing and understanding the gestures and facial expression Marty used to augment his words as well as the words he used. I found that if I was in tune with how he was feeling, I could more easily piece together what he was telling me. Becoming a part of his unfolding story put us on the same page and would influence many of my decisions regarding what to do and when to do it. It was difficult to hear Marty's side of the story with his family so involved in our sessions – there seemed to be an overwhelming amount of chaos in the family narratives, and it was clear that they did not see potential for improvement (Hamilton, 2018).

As my work with Marty and his family progressed, it dawned on me that the highly supportive nature of the family and the roles family members were playing were resulting in Marty being cared for but risked him not being empowered to work hard on his rehabilitation. The success of the therapy required him to engage in the sessions we had together, and to practice speech exercises regularly throughout each day. His motivation for this seemed low, and his family's narrative regarding his future was perpetuating a fatalistic view that recovery may or may not just happen. His recovery of effective speech was reliant on his motivation to do his homework! A requirement for client motivation to act is central to many health interventions. Whilst some interventions are "done to" the person (e.g., facial massage) or "done for" the person (e.g., computer software support application), much work requires action on the part of the person. This action, or health behavior, may be to augment remedial therapy sessions (as with the work I was doing with Marty), for lifestyle changes to promote health and wellbeing, or new learning as part of adjusting to acquired or developing disability.

Appreciating the client's motivation for health behavioral change is helpful for making decisions related to intervention strategies and models of service provision. There are several useful models that focus on client motivation for change. Although they were developed primarily for health promotion, I find that viewing the person through a theoretical model deepens my

understanding of their motivation and therefore likely participation in the therapy process. Two that have been useful to me are the Health Beliefs Model (HBM) (Rosenstock et al., 1988) and the Transtheoretical Model of Change (DiClemente & Prochaska, 1998).

The HBM was originally articulated in the 1950s (Champion & Skinner, 2008) to inform health promotion services. The model explores an individual's beliefs about the influence they have over their health and therefore their motivation to engage in health-enhancing behavior. It explores the demographic or contextual factors that influence the person's health behavior (e.g., ethnicity, cultural factors, socio-economic status, education, etc.), their perceptions about how severe the health issue is and how susceptible they are (termed "threat perception") and their likelihood for change based on their perception of benefits for and barriers to engaging in the health behavior.

For my work with Marty, the HBM guided me to explore cultural elements that might be affecting the family's collective response to Marty's accident. To better understand the cultural context, I decided to discuss my situation with a member of the rehabilitation team from the same ethnic background as Marty. This cultural supervision session helped me appreciate the importance Marty's mother would place on caring for him and helped me see things from a perspective unfamiliar to me. The HBM also considers the client's self-efficacy (belief that a future action is within one's capabilities) and cues for action (such as from media or educational material from a health professional) as influential on the likelihood of action. I hoped that helping Marty and his family understand the value of working on communication to ameliorate likely negative impacts on his future social function would be cues for action. I surmised that including the family in the intervention phase would enhance self-efficacy and help create a collective shift from their compensatory approach to one of remediation. Whilst the HBM was developed for use in health promotion services, considering the elements in terms of Marty and his community enhanced my understanding of their responses to and engagement with the work we were doing together.

Another model that I have found useful in understanding behavioral change is the Transtheoretical Model of Change (DiClemente & Prochaska, 1998). The developers propose that health behavior change involves progress through five specific stages of change: precontemplation, contemplation, preparation, action, and maintenance. Research into this model has shown that intervention that targets the specific stage of change the person is at is more effective than following generic intervention pathways. The conversations I had held with Marty and his family indicated that collectively they were in the contemplation stage regarding engaging in remedial work. They were considering therapy but other than attending appointments, were not engaged. I hypothesized that using this approach with the family unit might of itself be a cue for change and facilitate a shift toward active engagement in therapy. Additionally, using the Transtheoretical Model of Change throughout the intervention process would enhance the client–therapist relationship through demonstrating awareness of where Marty and family are at regarding health behavior change, and enhance our capacity for shared decision making. My comfort with MI would be helpful as this is a particularly good fit with the Transtheoretical Model of Change.

My focus now was to facilitate a shift from the current model of Marty being cared for by his family to working toward restoration of skill. This necessitated my sharing the expertise I have and tapping into the wealth of knowledge and experience Marty and his family held.

SHARED EXPERTISE

Both practitioner and client bring specific specialist knowledge to the decisions to be made. The person has knowledge of themselves and their unique circumstances, history, contextual factors, and an understanding of what might or might not work best for them. The practitioner, however, has an understanding of best practice in terms of research evidence (with an associated responsibility to translate this for clients), the resources available to them and the client, what they can offer in terms of skills and expertise, and an understanding of intervention, progress, and prognosis. This illustrates the interrelatedness of the fingers on the FFF, where they all come together to form a whole.

In my setting, I understood that I have practice responsibility and therefore must provide information and articulate choices I can offer so Marty is well informed prior to consenting to intervention and selecting from options available. Whilst working out how to do this with Marty and his extended family, I started to focus on the "thumb" part of the framework and think about my reasoning. Situating myself as expert and expecting Marty to consent to my intervention suddenly seemed contrary to person-centered practice, as the power differential was uncomfortably evident to me. The realignment of power integral to genuine person-centeredness was a challenge in the structure of the system I was embedded in. Whilst I could not change the system, this insight prompted me to negotiate the conversation with heightened sensitivity toward and respect for the position Marty and his family were in.

Through my prior experience, I had developed a good understanding of best practice intervention for the communication issues Marty presented with. As well as doing a thorough health condition analysis of CVA, I had read research evidence regarding overall intervention and specific speech language therapy for this population. I had a repertoire of evidence-based strategies and a cupboard full of resources. My decision at this point was regarding what knowledge I needed to share with Marty, and what choices I could provide him with for our work together. I knew that effective client education involves ensuring that I deliver relevant information that is both timely and able to be absorbed by the client. Everyone learns differently, so talking through material may work for some, others learn better through reading, observing, or experiencing. Many health conditions also influence people's capacity for new learning and may change what learning strategies are useful (Braungart et al., 2019). Through a humanistic lens, attention to emotions and the relationship between the practitioner (teacher) and client (learner) is paramount. The practitioner acts as a facilitator of learning; the client in whom the learning is situated comprehends what has been learned. The practitioner therefore must be able to provide information in a manner that is in tune with the person's emotional state (is this the best time for education or should my approach be supportive?) and their capacity for learning. Equally important is that the information has a direct link with their goals and is in tune with their attitudes and beliefs.

To maximize potential for learning, consideration should also be given to the immediate demands of the environment (should I see Marty at home, with his children around, or in my clinic room?) and to the phase of the client's current episode of care (my information sharing at intervention phase would differ from my initial assessment phase and will change again at the time of discharge).

Despite having explained to Marty and his family the rationale behind the exercises I was encouraging, it was difficult to know exactly what new understanding had been constructed by him. A constructivist approach to teaching and learning means that I need to scaffold or layer information so that Marty and his family can build on their understanding, and I need to ensure the information is immediately relevant for their current needs. So, telling them about the whole of the intervention road ahead might have been overwhelming whilst coming to terms with the extent of the communication issues, but it will become relevant once we are under way and planning for gradual reduction in service. This staged approach to client education would work well when viewed through the Transtheoretical Model of Change – my initial approach was to assist Marty to move toward the action stage in terms of engagement with therapy.

As I grappled with understanding Marty's reticence for engagement in rehabilitation, I thought more about what impacts on learning. Although born in this country, he had grown up with strong cultural role models. Social Learning Theory (Bandura 1977 cited in Braungart et al., 2019) helps me appreciate the automatic way we develop and adjust our beliefs and behaviors to fit with the world around us. My developing relationship with Marty and his family, and my cultural supervision session, influenced my perception of why things were as they were for Marty. This reinforced the premise in person-centered practice that one cannot know how to engage with an individual until engagement with the individual has begun. However, it occurred to me that most sessions had been with Marty and family members. Perhaps in my eagerness to be family inclusive, I had done Marty a disservice. I had missed a decision point that should have sat squarely in my palm – how to negotiate family-centeredness and individual therapy. My supervisor agreed.

I called Marty offering an individual session in my office which he willingly accepted. That session was profoundly useful for both of us. In his halting way (as he still had word-finding difficulties), Marty shared how torn between the two cultures he has always been, and how difficult it is for him to fit in with family expectations as well as with wider societal norms. He appreciated that his mother needed to take care of him, and he equally appreciated his need to work toward regaining his independence. This was a profoundly helpful addition to the narrative Marty and his family had been sharing, and illustrated his envisaged future being that of restitution, quite different from the chaos he was currently experiencing (Hamilton, 2018). As a result of this session, we agreed he would have structured therapy sessions with me in my office, and that I would occasionally see him with his family. This seemed like a sensible way to manage working with Marty and maintaining my connection with the family. I felt more confident we could get the work done and Marty seemed to have moved into the action stage.

I needed to draft a report justifying my request for more hours to spend with Marty and sought the multidisciplinary team's input. I discovered that the occupational therapist considered Marty to be a long way off being ready for return to work. I was initially surprised – Marty's expressive aphasia was mild compared with many clients I had worked with and had improved over the last six weeks. His facial muscles were stronger and his speech was easier to understand. However, in conversation with the occupational therapist, I became aware of the need for a more sophisticated level of communication in his role of manager, including written communication and presentations using PowerPoint. These were exceedingly difficult for Marty. Whilst I had taken a bio-psycho-social approach and had a comprehensive focus on client goals in terms of function in the home and social environment, I had failed to ascertain goals to meet the rest of Marty's everyday life, especially return to work (Forsgren et al., 2022).

I thought about what I had done and why – usually my use of reflective practice is in the moment, "reflecting in practice," and I do not usually write a reflection. This time, to help with preparation of my report, I wrote following Gibb's Model of Reflection (Gibbs, 1988) and found the process humbling and insight provoking. Despite my best efforts to "know the client" and their goals and needs, my intervention decisions were overly influenced by my past experience with CVA. The outcomes I had measured were related to speech, not other elements of communication, and I had subconsciously used my usual client population (retirees) as a benchmark. I had also not sought input from Marty in terms of outcomes measurement – my measures were all important but objective. This was another example of the power differential – my professional views regarding outcomes were dominant. I talked about this with some of my colleagues and learned about Patient-reported Outcomes and Patient-reported Outcome Measures (Weldring & Smith, 2013), and about the concept of routine outcomes measurement. There are numerous tools designed for individual disciplines to enable the client voice in outcomes measurement, so I resolved to find one for speech language therapy and implement it in my practice.

When looking for an outcome measure that would enable me to adjust sessions based on Marty's perspective, I found literature on feedback-informed treatment (FIT) which advocates soliciting feedback from the client on a sessional basis. The feedback is used to adjust intervention in the next session (Miller et al., 2015). The developers report that adjusting aspects of intervention that are not working for the client strengthens the client–therapist alliance and enhances client motivation, leading to better client engagement and outcomes, and more tailored intervention plans by the therapist. Although developed with talk-based therapies in mind, the principles of FIT can be used in any health intervention.

I had always valued feedback from peers and my supervisor, and consciously used this for professional development, integrating this into the use of self (thumb) part of the FFF. However, client feedback had been limited to feedback forms completed at the end of the episode of care or spontaneous expressions from clients expressing how they felt about therapy. My professional practice would benefit if I sought and responded to regular immediate feedback from clients. Two brief rating scales are advocated for use in FIT – the Session Rating Scale (Miller et al., 2002) and Outcome Rating Scale (Miller & Duncan, 2000). I could see how they would be valuable for many of my clients with some adaptation required because of the nature of communication issues experienced by clients of speech language therapy. I surmised that the use of feedback from Marty after each session from the beginning of our relationship would have provided opportunities for him to express needs from a broader perspective.

This reflection led me to notice the lack of client-centered tools in our service; assessment strategies could easily include ascertaining the person's perspective, as forms that document goals and intervention plans could provide prompts for the clients' views. We were directed to write SMART (specific, measurable, achievable, realistic, timebound) goals so simply adding SMARTER (shared, monitored, accessible, relevant, transparent, evolving, and relationship-centered) (Hersh et al., 2012) would make a real difference! Embarking on this critical thinking process helped me appreciate how I had assumed that the established workplace culture was an appropriate structure for me; however, it did not enable person-centered practice as much as it could. I resolved to advocate some changes that would make the client's perspective more embedded in our service (Figure 5.1, Table 5.1).

"Person-centred care is holistic, flexible, creative, personal, and unique. Person-centred care is not reductionist, standardized, detached, and task based. Not unless the person wants it to be" (Evardsson, 2015, p. 66).

This chapter has emphasized the importance of keeping the person or people receiving our service front of mind and treating them as partners in the professional reasoning process. A collaboration that is formed from a strong therapeutic relationship and built on sharing expertise and decisions will enhance outcomes for the people we work with. The contextual factors that surround the practice and the client are also influential in professional reasoning, are situated on the fourth finger of the framework and explored in the following chapter.

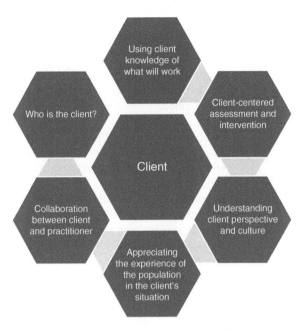

FIGURE 5.1   The client perspective in the Five Finger Framework for professional reasoning.

TABLE 5.1   Key Points

Role	Key Points
Practitioner/ student	Who is the client? Ascertain who the stakeholders are and those who are direct clients. • The person presenting. • The funder/insurer. • The family/significant others. • The parents/caregivers. • The community or group. Learn about the client group or population. • Attend conferences with service user presentations. • Internet-based resources where client narratives and views are available, e.g., Database of Individual Patients' Experiences. • Connect with support groups, client advocates, people with lived experience. Learn about the client. • Incorporate room for the client perspective in the assessment phase. • Health condition analysis using the International Classification of Function (ICF). • Consider age and stage of life. • Culture and ethnicity. • Values, beliefs, goals, and what the client wants from the intervention.

(Continued)

TABLE 5.1   (Continued)

Role	Key Points
	<ul><li>Socio-economic and education level factors.</li><li>Barriers and enablers to accessing and participating in intervention.</li><li>Use cultural supervision.</li><li>Social determinants of health (e.g., economic stability, education, health and healthcare, neighborhood and built environment, social support and community context).</li></ul>Relationship first.<ul><li>Therapeutic communication.</li><li>Therapeutic use of self.</li><li>Mindfulness training to be present with the client.</li><li>Use opportunities to meet with clients – groups, support groups, etc.</li><li>Some standard phrases that help you maintain professional boundaries.</li><li>Objectivity.</li><li>Managing uncomfortable relationships.</li><li>Focus on the job at hand.</li><li>Maintain professional boundaries.<ul><li>Personal disclosures.</li><li>Conscious use of self.</li><li>Safety.</li></ul></li></ul>Collaboration.<ul><li>Individualized goal setting.</li><li>Feedback-informed treatment or other ways of collecting and responding to client feedback.</li><li>Provide education/information to enable participation and choice.</li><li>Use choice as much as possible.</li><li>Client engagement is a good predictor of outcomes.</li><li>Incorporate tools that enable person-centered practice – assessment, feedback-informed treatment.</li></ul>
Manager	Shared expertise.<ul><li>Ensure assessments that are standard for the service are limited and there is space for assessment to be related to the situation and need of the individual.</li><li>Participatory management style.</li><li>Work with service users and families to develop protocols and guidelines and processes for the service.</li></ul>Who is the client?<ul><li>Awareness of the culture of the workplace in terms of relationships with clients.</li><li>Manage processes to ensure all stakeholders are appropriately considered.</li><li>Provide opportunities for cultural awareness and supervision.</li><li>Analyze the community to inform staff of factors that determine client base – socio-economics, ethnicities, access to services, urban–rural mix, health, and wellbeing issues most addressed by the service.</li></ul>

TABLE 5.1 (Continued)

Role	Key Points
	Develop networks with other service providers. • Select and use a framework for helping staff understand the client population, e.g., Social Determinants of Health Framework. Relationship first. • Provide resources and training on therapeutic relationship building and maintenance. • Have mentors of good person-centered practice for inexperienced staff to access and observe. Collaboration. • Incorporate a client-centered approach in service policies and guidelines. • Include client voice in service planning and development. • Utilize client advisors.
Educator	Shared expertise. • Ensure outcomes measurement that are based on client perspective as well as objective measures are taught. • Patient-reported Outcomes Measurement. • Routine outcomes measurement tools, e.g., feedback-informed treatment. Who is the client? • Use resources that provide students with content from individuals with lived experience – YouTube, Ted Talks, podcasts. • Invite guest speakers from service user community. • Ensure students understand sociopolitical complexities that influence person-centered practice. • Link education regarding cultural sensitivity to working in a person- or group-centered way. Relationship first. • Emphasize, teach, and role model relationship building, maintenance, and repair skills. • Use a relationship teaching model, e.g., Intentional Relationship Model (Taylor, 2020). Collaboration. • Consider "doing with" and "not doing to" as a threshold concept for students to cross. • Give students opportunities to see it in action. • Ensure students learn how to effectively help clients learn. • Feedback skills – giving and receiving.
Supervisor	• Use FFF to guide supervision sessions. • Structure supervision session to encourage depth. • Maintain awareness of supervisee's perception of client situation. • Help supervisee maintain awareness of their own beliefs and values.

REFERENCES

Baldwin, S. A., Wampold, B. E., & Imel, Z. E. (2007). Untangling the alliance-outcome correlation: exploring the relative importance of therapist and patient variability in the alliance. *Journal of Consulting and Clinical Psychology, 75*(6), 842.

Braungart, M. M., Braungart, R. G., & Gramet, P. R. (2019). Applying learning theories to healthcare practice. In S. Bastable (Ed.), *Nurse as educator: Principles of teaching and learning for nursing practice* (pp. 69–111)). Jones and Bartlett Learning.

Champion, V. L., & Skinner, C. S. (2008). The health belief model. In K. Glanz, B. Rimer, & K. Viswanath (Eds.), *Health behavior and health education: Theory, research, and practice* (pp. 45–65). John Wiley & Sons.

DiClemente, C. C., & Prochaska, J. O. (1998). Toward a comprehensive, transtheoretical model of change: stages of change and addictive behaviors. In W. R. Miller & N. Heather (Eds.), *Treating addictive behaviors* (pp. 3–24). Plenum Press.

DIPex International. (2023). `https://dipexinternational.org/`

Edvardsson, D. (2015). Notes on person-centred care: what it is and what it is not. *Nordic Journal of Nursing Research, 35*(2), 65–66.

Forsgren, E., Åke, S., & Saldert, C. (2022). Person-centred care in speech-language therapy research and practice for adults: a scoping review. *International Journal of Language & Communication Disorders, 57*(2), 381–402.

Gibbs, G. (1988). *Learning by doing: A guide to teaching and learning methods.* Further Education Unit.

Hamilton, T. B. (2018). Narrative reasoning. In B. A. Boyt Schell & J. W. Schell (Eds.), *Clinical and professional reasoning* (pp. 171–202). Wolters Kluwer.

Hersh, D., Worrall, L., Howe, T., Sherratt, S., & Davidson, B. (2012). SMARTER goal setting in aphasia rehabilitation. *Aphasiology, 26*(2), 220–233.

Mattingly, C., & Hayes Fleming, M. (2019). Action and narrative: two dynamics of clinical reasoning. In J. Higgs, G. M. Jensen, S. Loftus, & N. Christensen (Eds.), *Clinical reasoning in the health professions* (pp. 119–127). Elsevier.

Meyer, J., & Land, R. (2003). *Threshold concepts and troublesome knowledge: Linkages to ways of thinking and practising within the disciplines.* University of Edinburgh.

Miller, S. D., & Duncan, B. L. (2000). *Outcome rating scale.* Authors.

Miller, S. D., Duncan, B. L., & Johnson, L. (2002). *Session rating scale.* Authors.

Miller, S. D., Hubble, M. A., Chow, D., & Seidel, J. (2015). Beyond measures and monitoring: realizing the potential of feedback-informed treatment. *Psychotherapy, 52*(4), 449.

Miller, W. R., & Rollnick, S. (2012). *Motivational interviewing: Helping people change.* Guilford Press.

Rogers, C. R. (1986). Carl Rogers on the development of the person-centered approach. *Person-Centered Review, 1*(3), 257–259.

Rosenstock, I. M., Strecher, V. J., & Becker, M. H. (1988). Social learning theory and the health belief model. *Health Education Quarterly, 15*(2), 175–183.

Sackett, D. L., Straus, S. E., Richardson, W. S., Rosenberg, W., & Haynes, R. B. (2000). *Evidence-based medicine: How to practice and teach EBM* (2nd ed.). Churchill Livingstone.

Taylor, R. R. (2020). *The intentional relationship: Occupational therapy and use of self.* F.A. Davis.

Vahdat, S., Hamzehgardeshi, L., Hessam, S., & Hamzehgardeshi, Z. (2014). Patient involvement in health care decision making: a review. *Iranian Red Crescent Medical Journal, 16*(1), e12454.

Weldring, T., & Smith, S. M. (2013). Article commentary: Patient-reported outcomes (pros) and patient-reported outcome measures (PROMs). *Health Services Insights, 6*, HSI–S11093.

CHAPTER 6

Knowing the Context like the Back of Your Hand

Contextual Influences on Professional Reasoning

Helen Jeffery

Principal Lecturer, School of Occupational Therapy, Te Pūkenga|Otago Polytechnic, New Zealand

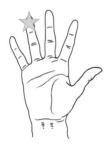

INTRODUCTION

It is important to consider the broad perspective of the often unseen elements of the environment that affect practice. Environment, the fourth finger in the Five Finger Framework (FFF), refers to (a) the practice environment (work setting), (b) the community in which the setting is situated, and (c) the client's home and cultural environment.

Knowledge from research and other literature is integrated into service provision through development and use of protocols, clinical guidelines, and structures that support good practice. This knowledge translation ideally establishes how best practice guidelines and research evidence can form local best practice. Many of these decisions are now made locally to match the needs of that particular population.

The culture of the team and the service guidelines impact reasoning and decision making through how work is distributed, workflow is structured, and the relationships and community that are established in the workplace. Additionally, a collective understanding of health often forms within or is guided by service settings and influences reasoning. Workplaces are resourced differently, and access to these resources needs to be factored into local decision

Professional Reasoning in Healthcare: Navigating Uncertainty Using the Five Finger Framework, First Edition.
Edited by Helen Jeffery, Linda Robertson, Jan Hendrik Roodt, and Susan Ryan.
© 2024 John Wiley & Sons Ltd. Published 2024 by John Wiley & Sons Ltd.

making. Materials and equipment required for certain interventions may or may not be available, time allocation for intervention differs depending on funding structures and workflow processes, and allocation of human resources affects professional decisions regarding how much to offer or options for multidisciplinary input.

The culture of the local community has implications for professional reasoning processes. Factors such as ethnicity, urban or rural, and lower or higher socioeconomic status of groups influence decisions in terms of interventions that are available and appropriate. Communities that are multicultural have a different flavor from those that have less ethnic diversity, large inner-city services often operate vastly differently from isolated and rural settings, and financial resources of the setting and within the broader community affect what is possible to offer. Availability of community resources influences decisions regarding community engagement and participation, and service delivery is influenced by the nature of the community, such as home visits versus client attending a clinic, group work versus individual work, specialization versus generic work, and multidisciplinary work versus interdisciplinary work.

This finger focuses on the question "How do I do things here, in this place, and what can help me ascertain this?" and encourages consideration of all these contextual elements as an integral part of professional reasoning.

Setting the Scene

I am a social worker with two years' experience working in a large general hospital, covering the surgical wards. I have recently moved to work in a small inner-city community youth service called One Stop that operates as a "one stop shop." Young people can self-refer and services offered include sexual health, general health issues including mental health, and social issues such as homelessness or family violence. We are a multidisciplinary team and take it in turns being on duty at the front desk to help people access the professional or service they need in that moment. We do have a caseload management system which helps provide consistency in terms of our client base. When not on duty, we work with people spontaneously as they arrive and have scheduled follow-up appointments with clients we are working with closely. We also have an outreach service, where we agree to meet clients in the community or at their home if there are risk factors. Sometimes other services work with us, such as the police, community agencies, etc. Keira is 17 years old from a family that has been struggling with poverty, unemployment, and domestic violence.

When I started work at One Stop, I had a four-week orientation to the service and community. This seemed excessive when I began – a whole month just to get an understanding of the service! I questioned my supervisor about this, and she explained that I would constantly need to make decisions about what to do when working with the young people and that the team uses the Five Finger Framework (Jeffery et al., 2021) to help with their individual and collective decision making. She talked about one of the "fingers" being context or environment and explained that the impact of the local community culture and resources has a significant effect on what we can decide to do (Smith & Higgs, 2019). She reminded me of the concept of pragmatic reasoning, "the aspect of reasoning that therapists use to attend to the practical realities of service delivery" (Boyt Schell, 2018, p. 204).

One month on and I have found that the orientation in terms of context has been profoundly helpful for my professional decision making. I have learned the benefits of intentionally thinking about the context in three ways, identified by Ryan and Higgs (2008) as *thinking wide* (social, political, and legislative context), *thinking about the community context* (service, facilities, and client base) and *thinking about the service structure* (resources and location). This has helped me appreciate the benefits of knowing the wider community as well as my workplace and through the lens of the population I would be working with.

COMMUNITY CONTEXT: SERVICES

Although I had lived here for some years and had social and recreational pursuits in the local community, I had not worked as a social worker in the community and had not been involved in the youth community. My last job at the hospital was vastly different; there, the clients were all in the same place (hospital ward), and appointments made with family were in the ward as well. There were clinical guidelines and treatment protocols established to assist staff in making appropriate decisions in specific situations (Taylor, 2000). For most admissions, there was a clear process through to discharge and my role was distinct, the multidisciplinary team understood what I did, and our professional boundaries were clear to each other and to the clients. That job had helped me develop a strong professional identity as a social worker, which was reinforced by

how others saw me and what they expected of me. This new job was such a big shift in focus that although I felt confident that my social work identity was a good match, I initially felt overwhelmed. Thanks to the longer orientation phase, this feeling was reduced by the end of the first month.

My orientation in this job included night watches with the community police, where I drove around the city with them and observed their interactions with young people. They showed me places where young people congregated at night and talked about different areas of the city and the struggles of people living in poverty. They helped me understand the primary alcohol and substance use issues for young people as they saw it on the streets and in the parks, and the typical behaviors that were often problematic. I also learned about places young people spent time in that were safer, the environments they accessed and activities they engaged in that supported healthy development and prosocial behavior. Importantly, they role modeled to me ways of communicating with young people. I was impressed with their deescalation skills and the rapport they established with the young people. I did witness some scenes that were confronting for me, including arrests, but even those situations helped me appreciate the wider environment as I was orientated to the systems and the cells!

The police spoke favorably of many community services that were available to young people. One was an outreach mental health service where I was able to shadow a nurse and observe his interactions with the homeless community, particularly those who took regular medications to help with their mental health challenges. The nurse explained that they worked closely with One Stop for their young people, but they also worked with people throughout the lifespan.

The importance of getting effective service in place for young people so that their trajectory in life could become safe and healthful was brutally evident to me through this experience. Time here and with other services helped me understand what they did, how they did it, their funding and staffing, and how they linked with One Stop. They were all aware of One Stop and spoke of how they supported young people to access our service, and their perspective on what was particularly valuable about our service.

As I spoke with the people in these services, I felt part of a city-wide network with the common goal of youth health and wellbeing at the heart of it. These experiences helped me understand that I was being socialized into the community of practice that existed around working with young people in this place and time. A community of practice is a group of people who interact regularly to learn from each other about a shared concern or area of passion (Wenger et al., 2002), and includes formal and informal structures. I was told about a gathering of people in the city who work with young people in the social and healthcare sectors. They meet every two months, take turns to present and facilitate discussion groups based on the presentation. It sounded fantastic – attending and contributing would enable me to use the full range of knowledge and skills of social work and belong to a likeminded community that would challenge and enhance my practice.

COMMUNITY CONTEXT: CULTURAL

I know that culture is in part about social behavior and the norms that are established by and in populations, as well as ethnicity. We live in a country colonized by the British

and in more recent years populated also by people from many parts of the world. The resultant diversity in the multicultural context of the city is vibrant and interesting. I had always loved going to the Saturday market where this cultural diversity is brought to life through the crafts, art, food, and music on offer.

However, my orientation to the city services was confronting as I became aware of the more hidden issues and social challenges – the areas of poverty and the impact that has on how communities survive was particularly confronting, and I realized the importance of considering clients' socio-economic position in professional reasoning. I saw services that supported refugees as they transitioned to our place and began to understand the depth of their trauma and how difficult their journey to their new home had been. Now they had to learn to get by in a completely new culture.

The concept of assimilation came to mind – how could these people navigate living in this new world and at the same time maintain their own cultural identity and ways of being? This is even more pertinent with the Indigenous population, who have experienced enforced assimilation and now suffer the associated disconnection from land, people, and culture, and experience fundamental health and wellbeing issues as a direct result of this disconnection. I was deeply aware of the Indigenous issues as they have affected my own family. My grandmother on my father's side is Indigenous, and as I grew up, I spent time with her and that side of my family. She and my great aunts and uncles helped me understand the history, cultural norms, and interconnectedness of everything in the natural world integral to many Indigenous cultures. This has helped me appreciate the importance of the natural environment, and the part we need to play in promoting sustainable practices and considering the health of the planet as integral to the health of people – it is becoming so important that I have heard it should become a natural component of professional reasoning for everyone (Hess & Rihtman, 2023). I heard a quote recently that has cemented this concept for me: "We abuse land because we regard it as a commodity belonging to us. When we see land as a community to which we belong, we may begin to use it with love and respect" (Leopold, A. cited in Beery et al., 2015, pp. 203–204). My family have also helped me understand culture from a collectivist perspective, where the collective or group takes precedence and where harmony within the collective is of the utmost importance (Turpin & Iwama, 2011). Being able to understand an individual's place and role in their group, and the importance of belonging, shifts the emphasis from person centered to a much broader perspective and must influence the reasoning that informs our professional decisions (Trentham et al., 2022; Turpin & Iwama, 2011).

This experience has also reinforced a deep appreciation of my privileged position in this community –a safe upbringing and a good education leading to a qualification that enables me to enjoy well-paid work have protected me from the hardship experienced by many of my people. I have been able to walk to a certain extent in both worlds but as most of my life experiences were within a Euro-centric worldview, I had developed an individualist perspective. I remember during my social work training learning about explicit and implicit bias and how practitioners' bias can have a negative impact on the service they provide (Restall & Egan, 2022). We completed an implicit bias assessment (Greenwald et al., 2011), so I made a note to do this again and to take it more seriously.

ORGANIZATIONAL CULTURE

I also spent time understanding and adjusting to the organizational culture of One Stop, vastly different from my last job. Organizational culture is defined by Pandit (2020) as "the underlying beliefs, assumptions, values and ways of interacting that contribute to the unique social and psychological environment of an organisation. Culture also includes the organisation's vision, values, norms, systems, symbols, language, assumptions, beliefs and habits" (p. 1). While I had read the values and mission statement for One Stop, it was through observation and interaction with others that I truly began to appreciate the culture.

One such crucial observation was what happens in the social room – a space open to any young person wanting to pop in. The staff on duty there kept an eye on what was happening, welcomed new people, and offered them snacks and juice. They were hosts as much as anything but the more I watched, the more I saw assessment and care happening. The only criteria for young people to attend were that they register with the service and commit to some shared values which included nonviolent behavior and communication. I saw staff smoothly manage young people who arrived intoxicated, distressed, or hungry. Different staff had distinct roles, and although these were well established and clients were well matched with the appropriate discipline for individual care, in the social room the work was generic. Here I began to understand a part of the clients' journey with One Stop, and how intake, assessment, and appointments were initiated – all influential on professional reasoning.

One Stop also provides safe socialization activity-based groups through the week, and I took a turn at cofacilitating the drop-in group. This is an open fun group where food is available and the young people are in contact with each other and with staff. Here, they can quietly say if they want to have an appointment.

I noticed a young woman, Keira, who attended the session but spent most of her time on the periphery. I offered her a soft drink, sat with her and in chatting learned a little about her family. Her father was of European descent and her mother came from an Indigenous family. Her father had been violent and engaged in criminal activity and had been imprisoned when Keira was 11 years old. Keira's mother provided as best she could for the five children, and the home was more settled once the influence of her father was removed. I shared a little about myself, where I came from and found some common ground with Keira as I knew that connections and relationship are important with everyone, but especially so in our Indigenous community. Our capacity to be able to include cultural elements into professional reasoning develops over time and in stages. Cultural responsiveness is about being able to deliver healthcare that is congruent with the client's cultural beliefs and practices, and is reliant on cultural awareness, knowledge, and safety (Simpson & Cox, 2019). My connection with Keira was in part enabled by my capacity to incorporate aspects of my cultural knowledge and safety into what I considered to be important in my communication with her – these elements are all part of use of self (thumb).

SERVICE PROCESSES

The next week, I observed an initial assessment so that I could learn about some of the processes and structures in the service. The client was Keira, who presented somewhat unkempt and anxious, but she visibly relaxed when I entered the room. The connection we had already formed was helpful for both of us. As I listened to the interview, I noticed how much it seemed like a gentle conversation, and not at all like the initial assessments I had been part of in other work environments. We gradually uncovered the level of need in Keira's circumstances – she was estranged from her family and living with friends. She had no access to money and was using charity food banks. She was in a relationship with a young man living in the same place, who was helping her cope with her anxiety, low mood, and sense of despair through sharing his drugs with her. Keira spoke in a quiet and hesitant manner and after about 20 minutes made it clear she did not want to stay. My colleague supported her choice to leave the interview and encouraged her to come back to drop-in groups whenever she wanted to.

After Keira left, we filled in the form and I was surprised at how much information we had managed to gather, and the extent of detail required on the documentation. My colleague showed me the processes for filing electronic records and the policy related to documentation and care pathways, and talked through the suite of assessment tools we had access to. Knowing what is usual to use and what other tools are available meant I would not struggle when making assessment decisions. I had been shown where written protocols were stored; there were protocols for almost any eventuality and I had been given time to read them and talk with my supervisor about them. Many of these protocols linked directly to research evidence; my supervisor helped me appreciate that protocols, care guidelines, even group session plans were all evidence based, and the team met annually to ensure the evidence they were incorporating into their systems and interventions reflected best practice. This organizational support for evidence-based practice was evident in many diverse forms and made it easier to put research into practice (Bennett et al., 2016).

There is a specific model the service uses, based on a social model of health, and I could see already how the collective use of this model helped the staff work together and find common ground. Importantly, I was able to see the parameters of what I could and could not offer in this environment in terms of service and intervention – the decisions I would need to make on a day-to-day basis would draw from all this contextual knowledge.

TEAM CULTURE

The team met at the beginning of each shift (morning and afternoon) to plan and allocate work as required. Poor communication is known to be a main feature of client dissatisfaction with services. This can be ameliorated by effective collaboration and communication between teams, team members, and clients, which enhances health service provision (Trede & Higgs, 2019). At these meetings, I witnessed collaborative transdisciplinary decision making, where the team members, through mutual respect, were able to discuss, negotiate, and come to decisions with relative ease. There was evidence of team relationships that support therapy processes and enable optimal practice within the team.

The following week at one of the meetings, the team leader told us that Keira had popped in and requested an appointment with me. The team discussed her situation and her request, agreed that social work was an appropriate approach and acknowledged that I was ready to engage with my first client on an individual basis. This discussion illustrated the work allocation process, the use of specialist skills inherent

in specific professions, the flow of the client journey through the service, and the associated allocation of staff and other resources. It is important to understand these factors when making decisions about what can be offered. The team seemed to especially endorse allocating Keira to work with me once I shared that I had a cultural connection with her; this connection influenced the decision of the team to entrust her care to me and would influence the approach I took with her. I was impressed that culture featured so strongly in their decision. I was also impressed with the team culture – I was reassured that I would be fully supported, that I would work alongside another therapist for the first few weeks, and that good supervision would be available. This supportive team culture would give me confidence to make my decisions, and to ask for guidance when required – I felt a professional confidence that would not have been possible in many teams I have heard about!

SUPPORTING EVIDENCE-BASED PRACTICE

Despite the contact I had had with Keira and the information gathered, I felt I had no idea what to do at our first appointment. Would I do another assessment? Fill in the gaps from the last one? Find an issue to focus on? Just get to know her more? I reflected on what I already knew about her and found myself visualizing her current living situation and her needs based on the assumptions I had made. This helped me recognize that I just needed to know her better and formed the basis of the next session. Here I ascertained that Keira was feeling very disconnected from her usual supports. She alluded to an underlying issue, but was shy about disclosing what it was. She did not stay long but I reassured her she could come to the social room whenever she wanted to. The next day she came in again, somewhat intoxicated, demanded to see me and when we met stated she was pregnant and what was I going to do about it? I felt uncomfortable – I did not know what to do and was frustrated that the colleague I was working with was not available for that session. These emotions guided my decision to help Keira calm down and to set a formal appointment for the next day. I was sure I could have done more with Keira in that moment. However, this bought me some time to tap into the expertise of some of my colleagues (expertise of others finger). This situation was very new for me.

On taking it to supervision, I first worked through my frustration at not having my knowledgeable colleague on tap – this was a practice reality that I needed to work with. I then learned a little more about the context finger of the FFF. There were already protocols established for Keira's situation. My supervisor reminded me that the use of research literature was influential in decision making and translating knowledge into protocols made this practical. She mentioned that the protocols developed were based on best practice, and through knowledge translation activities. Knowledge translation refers to "any activity or process that facilitates the transfer of high-quality evidence from research into effective changes in health policy, clinical practice, or products" (Lang et al., 2007, p. 335). Translating, or making sense of the literature, is complicated by many influencing factors such as the practitioners involved, the client, the context of the service, and the resources available. I had always thought of knowledge translation as being simply putting research findings into practice, so looking at it in this way helped me appreciate why it is sometimes difficult to just do what the research findings suggest.

My supervisor described a knowledge translation framework that put things into perspective. The framework considers:

"What should be transferred to decision makers (the message)? To whom should research knowledge be transferred (the target audience)? By whom should research knowledge be transferred (the messenger)? How should research knowledge be transferred (the knowledge-transfer processes and supporting communications infrastructure)? With what effect should research knowledge be transferred (evaluation)?" (Lavis et al., 2003, p. 222)

This workplace clearly supported best practice, with the manager subscribing to journals for us and ensuring that we maintain an evidence portfolio, thereby helping with knowledge transfer from research to practitioner (research and literature finger). I had already learned that my colleagues were highly experienced and knowledgeable and appreciated the supportive culture in the team enabling me to ask naive questions without embarrassment. Simply exploring the concept of knowledge translation in supervision reinforced for me the links between the fingers in the FFF – research literature, the client, the support and expertise of others, and of course the context. Importantly for me at this point, I was shown the clinical guidelines and flow chart developed for staff managing disclosure of pregnancy at One Stop. Clinical guidelines not only assist with decision making but also guide client education and collaboration, maintain focus on the purpose of the service, and enhance standards of care and use of expert knowledge through an easy-to-use format (Taylor, 2000).

One point of knowledge translation activities is to facilitate a positive change in behavior (of practitioner and/or client) in line with best current evidence (Scott et al., 2012). I knew from my previous job that it is very difficult as an individual practitioner to change practice in a large organization with established culture and processes. However, I had not appreciated the knowledge translation that had been happening in the background – now I was learning about the value of guidelines to inform a service. Knowledge translation activities for services include development of protocols, procedures, and clinical guidelines, development of educational resources for staff and clients, development of decision aids for clients, educational meetings and sessions for staff and for/with clients. The benefits include enhanced outcomes, enhanced professional practice, and more effective use of resources (Scott et al., 2012; Trevena & McCaffery, 2019).

I started to think critically about how to apply the guidelines in this situation with Keira. Critical thinking and reflective practice share metacognitive processes; this ensures that we think about our thinking and encourages purposeful thinking (Gambrill, 2012). I needed to explore my assumptions about drug taking, teenage pregnancy, and many other elements of Keira's lifestyle; it was all so different from my own experience and as a novice practitioner in this type of work, I did not have a lot of experience to draw from. Novice practitioners take longer to make professional decisions – their ability to see patterns is restricted because of limited stores of previous relevant experiences in memory, important cues are not readily recognized, and there are limited steps in problem solving – these all inhibit smooth deliberate practice (Carr & Shotwell, 2018). I needed to use my knowledge of the local best practice in this setting and deliberate on what my next step with Keira would be.

I was much better prepared for my next session with Keira. I had challenged some of my personal assumptions, helped by reading more broadly and by attending one of the Teen Mothers support group sessions which I had been invited to during my orientation. I understood what services were available to Keira, what her options were, and how we could support her. However, she did not arrive at her appointment. I felt disappointed as I had prepared so well, and I was somewhat concerned. She had a lot going on, and there were risks related to her current lifestyle and her health and wellbeing. I had not yet visited a young person at home but appreciated the protocol stating that I needed to have another staff member attend with me because of the unknown home environment. I felt the value of this protocol when I checked her address and realized it is in one of the lower socio-economic areas of the city, with high crime rates – I was thankful for the time I spent with the police who helped me appreciate this.

Despite the supportive team culture, Friday was always busy as the weekend service had been reduced following a funding cut. We did not have the resources available for me to visit Keira until Tuesday afternoon. This was an eye opener for me; I had developed an impression that we could provide whatever services we wanted, but a conversation with colleagues over lunch helped me appreciate that I had been sheltered from many of the harsh realities of practice in this service as I orientated. As people spoke, I understood the pressure behind their work, having to triage who to spend extra time with, constantly evaluating risk factors and allocating service based on need. One of the reasons for such a well-supported daily drop-in service was to be able to monitor many young people at arm's length, and step in with valuable practitioner time only when required.

Availability of time, money, and human resources is an element of pragmatic reasoning (Boyt Schell, 2018) that until now I had not needed to consider.

As I prepared to leave work at the end of my shift, I began to feel increasingly worried. I remembered how anxious Keira had looked, her tearfulness, her anger, and a sense of hopelessness. I had focused more on her situation and not so much on her mental health and had no idea if I should be concerned or not. At the last minute, I phoned the emergency mental health team, who informed me that they have already visited the house Keira lives in, have met with her in the past and so she knows them and they know a little about her. They assured me they would check in on her as they visited one of her housemates that evening. My knowledge of the broader context in terms of services available was certainly helpful.

CLIENT CONTEXT

Monday arrived, and I found an email from the mental health emergency team to say that they had assessed Keira and found her mood low but no evidence of immediate risk to self or others. The next day, we ascertained that Keira did not have a phone and so my colleague and I went to her address and thankfully we found that she was there. I was shocked when I came face to face with the reality of her home situation. Keira was living in a squatting situation. The house was boarded up with access through a large window, it was filthy inside, cold and damp, and there were several young people living there. There was evidence of considerable alcohol and drug use.

Keira was initially embarrassed and angry at us turning up, but she agreed to talk. We discussed her living situation, her pregnancy, and her use of substances to cope with her distress. Having such a clear picture of the reality of Keira's physical and social home environment completely changed my perception of the urgency of the situation. I decided in the moment to identify risk factors and begin to work with her to ameliorate some of the risk more carefully. I was concerned that she might not be safe to be left here, but equally aware that I could not remove her against her will and had no idea where she could go. As well as anxious, I felt unsure of myself and what action to take; this level of uncertainty, unfamiliarity, and awareness of risk makes professional decisions more difficult (Smith & Higgs, 2019).

Fortunately, my colleague sensed the state I was in and gently took control of the conversation. She smoothly ascertained risk factors of the drug-taking behaviors and poor living conditions and how they related to Keira and to the baby. We had some written resources to offer Keira, which outlined her options and the risks and benefits associated with each decision she needed to make regarding drug taking and the pregnancy. Whilst it did not cover anything different from what we had talked about, it would likely be helpful for her to go over the information again in her own time. This is an example of a knowledge translation tool (or decision aid) designed for the client to help them with the decision (Costanzo et al., 2019). Education is commonly used, but there is evidence that education alone does not always facilitate behavioral change. I could now appreciate the point of the support groups, the networking with wider community resources, and the value of the open-endedness of the service we provided – discharge came when the person no longer required our service. We left Keira on the understanding that she would come to One Stop later that week to continue our work.

LEADERSHIP

While I felt I was doing OK with Keira, I decided to present my work and reasoning at our monthly case presentation meeting. I was impressed at how these meetings are facilitated and enjoyed being part of a meeting with the service manager. I appreciated the impact of her leadership style on the team's culture and performance. Leadership here seemed to aim to look after the wellbeing of staff and I recognized the four components of a transformational leadership style. These are (1) intellectual stimulation (e.g., questioning assumptions, fostering creativity); (2) individualized consideration (e.g., accepting individual differences, supporting learning); (3) inspirational motivation (e.g., displaying enthusiasm, communicating expectations); and (4) idealized influence (e.g., reflecting own values, high ethical standards) (Backman, 2022, p. 289). The team uses the FFF to structure these meetings, helpful for focusing on professional decision making.

I provided an overview of Keira in this crucial and complicated life event. We sat with a hand drawn on a piece of paper and noted what I had considered in relation to each of the fingers. Best practice evidence related to teen pregnancy and alcohol and drug use had been integrated into the protocols and resources I had accessed. I had used resources within One Stop and had helped Keira access resources in the wider community – she had joined a support group for teenage mothers and had a mentor to help her reduce her alcohol and drug use. As a team, we explored broader safety issues for Keira, and talked about her home situation being a significant risk factor. The team began to question me about the client finger. I had formed a good relationship with Keira, she was clearly comfortable with me, and I felt she trusted me. I had ascertained her perspective in several ways

and worked collaboratively with her. I had supported her decision to keep the baby and found ways to enable her goal to stop using substances. What more could I do in terms of the client finger?

Here, the expertise of my team members helped me realize that, despite our shared culture and how that had benefited our relationship, I had not looked beyond Keira as an individual. Whilst I had an awareness of the importance of connection with family and her people, I had processed the information available to me through an individualist lens. There was a missed opportunity for Keira to potentially benefit from Indigenous practices and knowledge to help her through this situation. Importantly, my opportunity to consider her perspective through her cultural world view (Gilsenan et al., 2012) was lost as I allowed myself to remain embedded in the Eurocentric systems surrounding us. Appreciating cultural diversity should go beyond that but despite our best efforts, most of the service at One Stop was Eurocentric in orientation, and even for Indigenous clients Western knowledge was privileged (Rogers et al., 2019). This triggered an animated discussion between us all and to draw the meeting to a close once time was up, we decided to use the next journal club to explore this issue. I agreed to find a piece of literature (research and literature finger) that would help work out how to integrate this cultural knowledge into reasoning and decisions.

The journal club, usually held at lunch time, was our only time as a team when we had any real academic conversation. I had initially been skeptical of its benefit but quickly saw that even if the research being presented did not have immediate value to me, it certainly got me stimulated and thinking! We used a journal club model called TREAT (Tailoring Research Evidence and Theory) (Wenke et al., 2018) which helped with our engagement, as the model ensures the research presented is contextually relevant, relates to shared goals of the group, has academic input, and the meeting includes food!

After this meeting, my supervisor took me to one side and gave me the name of a person who could act as cultural supervisor for me. She pointed to the thumb on the drawing and suggested that using this supervision might enhance my own ability to integrate cultural sensitivity and knowledge into professional decisions, as well as help me in my work with Keira.

ENDING THE PROCESS

My work with Keira continued well and after a few weeks we mutually agreed she did not need to continue using the services of One Stop, although she knew the door was always open for her. One year later, Keira popped in to see me and show off her baby. She looked happy and healthy and reported she was living with her mum, and they are sharing the care of the baby. She was volunteering with an environmental group, enjoying vegetable gardening at the community gardens and the sense of belonging these connections provided her. I reflected on the fears I had had regarding Keira and our work – all seemed to be resolved, even the fear that she would end up dependent on our service! Once connections and relationships were established at home and in her community, she no longer needed ours. I took the opportunity to have Keira complete a final Patient-related Outcomes Measure (PROM) (Field et al., 2019). One Stop has developed a PROM which is helpful for individual client progress measurement, clinical decision making, improving client education and health awareness, service-wide outcomes, service audits, and ascertaining patterns in client issues and responses (Field et al., 2019).

Since seeing Keira last, the journal club I had facilitated where we explored "At the interface: Indigenous health practitioners and evidence-based practice" by Rogers et al. (2019) had developed into a small working group to develop culturally responsive practices, integrate Indigenous practices, and encourage more Indigenous practitioners into our service. Keira's engagement with environmentalism had also caused me to think deeply about this in my own life and reflect on the fact that it is perhaps a professional responsibility as well as personal – one people, one planet (Dunphy, 2014). I was bold enough to share these thoughts and was surprised at the positive reception from my colleagues. I felt immensely proud of this work and reflected on how I would never have had the confidence to lead such a group without the support of the work environment I was immersed in.

My ability to:

- understand and draw from all the resources available to me in this environment;
- work within the time constraints and manage the daily and weekly workflow;
- manage the systems and processes integral to the service;
- appreciate and network with the wider community;
- learn to navigate the cultural complexity in this situation;

had all helped me appreciate the importance of holding both a wide and a focused view of context and environment in professional decision making (Figure 6.1, Table 6.1).

This chapter has illustrated the immense value of appreciating the local environment (community and service)

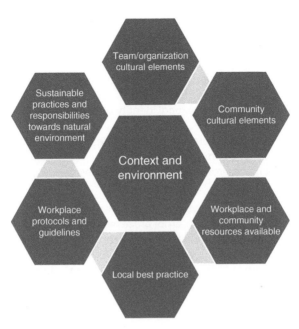

FIGURE 6.1   The context and environment perspective in the Five Finger Framework for professional reasoning.

TABLE 6.1   Key Points

Role	Key Points
Practitioner/student	• Learn about and connect with broader community. • Understand other services pertinent to the population you are working with. • Appreciate place of culture (including your own) in professional reasoning. • Take time to learn systems and use protocols and guidelines. • Orientate to the resources available in the community and within the service. • Use diversity of resources with clients for information sharing.
Educator	• Include the value of the broader community in relation to practice in teaching professional reasoning. • Emphasize the importance of culture as a key element in professional reasoning. • Implement an implicit and explicit bias tool with students. • Implement journal club with associated tools to support research evaluation. • Promote awareness of national policies and guidelines for best practice. • Emphasize and practice teamworking skills. • Facilitate interprofessional education opportunities – enhance professional identity and awareness of place in a multidisciplinary team.

(Continued)

TABLE 6.1   (Continued)

Role	Key Points
Supervisor	• Prompt supervisee to consider community environment and culture in professional reasoning. • Nurture professional identity and supervisee finding their place in the service. • Work on professional boundaries and safe ethical practice in diverse communities. • Ensure professional reasoning considers pragmatics of service provision.
Manager	• Comprehensive orientation for new staff – local community, services, and internal processes and systems. • Allow time for new staff to learn the ropes before full workload expected. • Enable flexibility in service provision to support cultural responsiveness. • Support involvement in community networks, e.g., support groups, communities of practice. • Enable maintenance of professional boundaries and identity. • Orientation to systems, policies, protocols, and resources. • Ensure protocols reflect best practice. • Have a knowledge translation system so best practice is enabled and adjusted with knowledge generation. • Enable discussion about and intentional work on effective team/service culture. • Promote positive team culture. • Enable routine academic knowledge-based interaction. e.g., journal club, in-service presentations, etc. • Limit workload for new staff as they learn to work in this setting. • Ensure resources are adequate for service.

when making professional decisions; some of the tools in Chapter 9 offer ideas for habitualizing consideration of the environment in reasoning. The extent to which the wider community influences practice decisions will vary depending on the profession and the workplace, but all services are situated within and influenced by the community they serve. Equally influential is the practice environment, represented by the team and service culture, the systems and supporting protocols and guidelines, and the extent to which practitioners are resourced and supported. Ideally, services incorporate best practice evidence into their protocols and guidelines, and through contextualizing the research evidence are able to formulate local best practice. This close relationship between practice settings and research literature justifies the position of the context finger next to the little finger, which represents research-based evidence and is covered in the next chapter.

REFERENCES

Backman, C. (2022). Leadership in occupational therapy. In M. Egan & G. Restall (Eds.), *Promoting occupational participation: Collaborative relationship-focused occupational therapy: 10th Canadian occupational therapy guidelines* (pp. 287–304). Canadian Association of Occupational Therapists.

Beery, T., Jönsson, K. I., & Elmberg, J. (2015). From environmental connectedness to sustainable futures: topophilia and human affiliation with nature. *Sustainability, 7*(7), 8837–8854.

Bennett, S., Allen, S., Caldwell, E., Whitehead, M., Turpin, M., Fleming, J., & Cox, R. (2016). Organisational support for evidence-based practice: occupational therapists perceptions. *Australian Occupational Therapy Journal, 63*(1), 9–18.

Boyt Schell, B. A. (2018). Pragmatic reasoning. In B. A. Boyt Schell & J. W. Schell (Eds.), *Clinical and professional reasoning* (pp. 203–223). Wolters Kluwer.

Carr, M., & Shotwell, M. P. (2018). Information processing theory and professional reasoning. In B. A. Boyt Schell & J. W. Schell (Eds.), *Clinical and professional reasoning* (pp. 73–104). Wolters Kluwer.

Costanzo, C., Doll, J., & Jensen, G. M. (2019). Shared decision making in practice. In J. Higgs, G. M. Jensen, S. Loftus, & N. Christensen (Eds.), *Clinical reasoning in the health professions* (pp. 181–190). Elsevier.

Dunphy, J. L. (2014). Healthcare professionals' perspectives on environmental sustainability. *Nursing Ethics, 21*(4), 414–425.

Field, J., Holmes, M. M., & Newell, D. (2019). PROMs data: can it be used to make decisions for individual patients? A narrative review. *Patient Related Outcome Measures, 10*, 233.

Gambrill, E. (2012). *Social work practice: A critical thinker's guide.* Oxford University Press.

Gilsenan, J. A., Hopkirk, J., & Emery-Whittington, I. (2012). Kai Whakaora Ngangahau – Māori occupational therapists' collective reasoning. In L. Robertson (Ed.), *Clinical reasoning in occupational therapy* (pp. 107–128). Blackwell Publishing.

Greenwald, T., Banaji, M., & Nosek, B. (2011). Project Implicit. https://implicit.harvard.edu/implicit/takeatest.html

Hess, K. Y., & Rihtman, T. (2023). Moving from theory to practice in occupational therapy education for planetary health: a theoretical view. *Australian Occupational Therapy Journal, 70*, 460–470.

Jeffery, H., Robertson, L., & Reay, K. L. (2021). Sources of evidence for professional decision-making in novice occupational therapy practitioners: clinicians' perspectives. *British Journal of Occupational Therapy, 84*(6), 346–354.

Lang, E. S., Wyer, P. C., & Haynes, R. B. (2007). Knowledge translation: closing the evidence-to-practice gap. *Annals of Emergency Medicine, 49*(3), 355–363.

Lavis, J. N., Robertson, D., Woodside, J. M., McLeod, C. B., & Abelson, J. (2003). How can research organizations more effectively transfer research knowledge to decision makers? *Milbank Quarterly, 81*(2), 221–248.

Pandit, M. (2020). Critical factors for successful management of VUCA times. *BMJ Leader.* https://bmjleader.bmj.com/content/5/2/121

Restall, G., & Egan, M. (2022). Collaborative relationship-focused occupational therapy. In M. Egan & G. Restall (Eds.), *Promoting occupational participation: Collaborative relationship-focused occupational therapy: 10th Canadian occupational therapy guidelines* (pp. 99–117). Canadian Association of Occupational Therapists.

Rogers, B. J., Swift, K., van der Woerd, K., Auger, M., Halseth, R., Atkinson, D., Vitalis, S., Wood, S., & Bedard, A. (2019). *At the interface: Indigenous health practitioners and evidence-based practice*. National Collaborating Centre for Aboriginal Health.

Ryan, S., & Higgs, J. (2008). Teaching and learning clinical reasoning. In J. Higgs, G. M. Jensen, S. Loftus, & N. Christensen (Eds.), *Clinical reasoning in the health professions* (3rd ed.). Elsevier, Butterworth-Heinemann.

Scott, S. D., Albrecht, L., O'Leary, K., Ball, G. D., Hartling, L., Hofmeyer, A., Jones, C., Klassen, T., Burns, K., Newton, A., Thompson, D., & Dryden, D. M. (2012). Systematic review of knowledge translation strategies in the allied health professions. *Implementation Science, 7*(1), 1–17.

Simpson, M. D., & Cox, J. L. (2019). Learning clinical reasoning across cultural contexts. In J. Higgs, G. M. Jensen, S. Loftus, & N. Christensen (Eds.), *Clinical reasoning in the health professions* (pp. 483–490). Elsevier.

Smith, M., & Higgs, J. (2019). Learning about factors influencing clinical decision making. In J. Higgs, G. M. Jensen, S. Loftus, & N. Christensen (Eds.), *Clinical reasoning in the health professions* (pp. 445–464). Elsevier.

Taylor, M. C. (2000). *Evidence-based practice for occupational therapists*. Wiley-Blackwell.

Trede, F., & Higgs, J. (2019). Collaborative decision making in liquid times. In J. Higgs, G. M. Jensen, S. Loftus, & N. Christensen (Eds.), *Clinical reasoning in the health professions* (pp. 159–168). Elsevier.

Trentham, B., Lalibert Rudman, D., Smith, H., & Phenix, A. (2022). The socio-political and historical context of occupational therapy in Canada. In M. Egan & G. Restall (Eds.), *Promoting occupational participation: Collaborative relationship-focused occupational therapy: 10th Canadian occupational therapy guidelines* (pp. 31–55). Canadian Association of Occupational Therapists.

Trevena, L., & McCaffery, K. (2019). Using decision aids to involve clients in clinical decision making. In J. Higgs, G. M. Jensen, S. Loftus, & N. Christensen (Eds.), *Clinical reasoning in the health professions* (pp. 191–200). Elsevier.

Turpin, M. J., & Iwama, M. K. (2011). *Using occupational therapy models in practice: A field guide*. Elsevier Health Sciences.

Wenger, E., McDermott, R., & Snyder, W. M. (2002). *Cultivating communities of practice*. Harvard Business School Press.

Wenke, R. J., Thomas, R., Hughes, I., & Mickan, S. (2018). The effectiveness and feasibility of TREAT (Tailoring Research Evidence and Theory) journal clubs in allied health: a randomised controlled trial. *BMC Medical Education, 18*(1), 1–14.

CHAPTER 7

Letting the Research Lend a Hand

Evaluating, Synthesizing, and Implementing Knowledges

Luciana Blaga[1] and Linda Robertson[2]

[1]Occupational Therapist, Te Whatu Ora|Health, New Zealand
[2]Associate Professor Emeritus, Occupational Therapy, Te Pūkenga, New Zealand

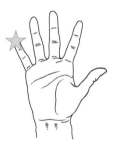

INTRODUCTION

Holding a foundation of science and established knowledge is an important element of professional reasoning and is emphasized in the use of principles of evidence-based practice (EBP). Research knowledge is situated on the little finger of the Five Finger Framework (FFF). This finger, while small, provides a point of balance in the hand and has an important role in hand strength, just as literature or research balances clinical decisions. This finger of the framework reminds practitioners to explore the potential and impact of utilizing best research evidence and ideas from bodies of knowledge to inform professional decision making. Here, the practitioner is asking "what is the research evidence base for this decision, how can the research and literature help me work out what to do and how to do it?"

Since the implementation of EBP, there has been a burgeoning of research in professional journals. The standards by which research should be judged as sufficient or relevant have also been targeted and explained in order that there is some consistency in the way that clinicians evaluate it. Not all research is equally robust and elements such as the context of the research, the views of the clients and the clinician's knowledge, expertise, and attitudes all have a significant impact on how relevant a particular study might be to a practice environment. Research involving participants will vary between countries and cultures – some studies cannot be translated from one community to another. However, these studies give ideas, and the use of the context finger will assist this process.

This chapter illustrates both the value of and some of the pitfalls involved in putting research findings into practice. Enablers and barriers to implementation of research findings, ways of accessing and ascertaining the relevance and trustworthiness of research, and the importance of holding the context in mind when considering what evidence to draw from are explored and illustrated through the narrative of a multidisciplinary team (MDT) working in a pain clinic. The scenario follows the team's experience of implementing a new program for managing persistent pain. The storyteller is a key member of the team who was aware of all elements. This illustrates that professional reasoning is often a collective process. Decisions that affect what services are provided, how resources are managed, service outcomes met and how teams work collaboratively all require deliberation and critical thinking at a team or group level.

The focus of this chapter is on the use of literature to inform the decisions that were made by the team and explores the professionals' role in collating and synthesizing evidence and then promoting a program that facilitates its use.

Setting the Scene

The exploration of reasoning reported in this chapter is related to sourcing and using literature to support a new program. The setting is a public hospital where a pain management team provides a service for people who have persistent pain. The team of five different health professionals (consultant, physiotherapist, clinical nurse, clinical psychologist, occupational therapist) has worked together over a six-year period. All members also have responsibilities in other clinical services, so are part time in their role with the pain management team. The scenario is the team's approach to providing a service to clients waiting for an appointment to see a pain consultant. On average, there is at least a four-month wait. The intention of the team was to provide an educational opportunity for these clients prior to their appointment with the consultant. This would introduce strategies that could assist them to manage their persistent pain. The reasoning of the interprofessional team when planning and evaluating the new service will be the focus in this scenario.

ABOUT THE SERVICE

Persistent pain is pervasive. It causes physical discomfort but also affects all aspects of life – work, social life, sleep, and, more generally, quality of life. Individuals experiencing this are on an ongoing quest for relief that is not always successful. Pain becomes their central focus and can result in loss of jobs, alienation of family and friends, isolation, feelings of frustration, and a sense of helplessness. Managing pain is complex and members of the team have found recent research that draws attention to the risk of promoting mainly passive biomedical treatment approaches (which are likely to increase need for and reliance on formal health services) as opposed to active self-management strategies (Davies et al., 2011b). A self-management approach is recognized as being central for high-quality integrated care where the focus is on improving function, controlling, and reducing the impact of pain rather than the total elimination of pain (Watson et al., 2014). This has prompted the team to explore strategies that could be introduced to enhance the service.

In this service, the process for clients receiving an appointment is as follows.

- Referrals received from the GPs or other specialists are triaged by the clinical pain nurse specialist in consultation with the team.
- Based on the points received in the triage process, each referral is placed on the waiting list for a two-hour MDT clinic appointment (this includes a pain consultant).
- Clients can then be offered sessions for more in-depth pain management strategies with one or more health team members (e.g., sleep management, relaxation strategies), or be discharged with advice.

Recently, there had been a reduction in access to pain consultants, resulting in fewer clinic numbers offered by this service. The team was frustrated by these circumstances because clients experienced long delays in being referred to health professionals who could assist them to manage their pain. This chapter explores the way in which this interprofessional team determined "best" practice in these circumstances and implemented a new approach to the management of a persistent pain service.

THE SEARCH TO DEVELOP A NEW APPROACH TO MANAGING THE PAIN SERVICE

The team was very interested in using a client self-management approach to their pain, thus removing the visit to the consultant. The potential of this approach had been reinforced by a conference presentation attended by two members of the team. A study presented by Australian clinicians appeared to be an ideal match between a proven method and the aspirations of the team. As the rest of the team listened to the summary of this presentation at an in-service education session, it was evident that they were excited as there were many similarities to their own ideas. At this point, there was no thought of looking for further approaches. To ensure that they had fully understood the ideas presented at the conference, the studies published on this project were located. This information enabled the team to check out details of how to set up a similar educational approach. The outcomes of the program were reported as reduced waiting times and increased use of active management strategies, ultimately resulting in greater patient satisfaction (Davies et al., 2011a). This was consistent with the desires of our team.

Motivated by the pragmatic consideration of staffing shortages combined with the realization that promising results were being reported by these other services in Australia using a preclinic education approach, the team was keen to trial something similar. By delivering essential information about pain management early, it was hoped that the waiting list would decrease and that clients would be more able to manage their pain symptoms. Therefore, it was decided that a new education program delivered prior to clients attending a first specialist assessment for pain management should be trialed. It was to be based on the work of Davies and her team (Davies et al., 2011b).

THE LITERATURE SEARCH

The team's question was: "What methods are being used in persistent pain management developments to improve services to their clients?" To explore this beyond the immediate source from the pain conference, the team decided that the following tasks were important.

- Identify literature related to programs that focus on managing persistent pain to discover the strength of the research and the key findings. Was there a Cochrane Review that summarized the research?
- To provide a reality check on issues that might need to be considered when developing the program, it was helpful to locate a team that had recently changed its approach to assisting people to manage persistent pain and consult them. What did they agree with in the research evidence and what did they query?
- Find out who has recently published in this area and locate articles, book chapters, and conference presentations by current researchers. On the assumption that these programs would be using the most up-to-date research, it would be a way of verifying the strength of previous findings and raising issues that might impact on the effectiveness of implementing a program in the service.
- Locate any literature that was based on client experiences. It was known that changing behavior related to pain management could be difficult. Based on client experience, what was essential to an effective program?
- Identify any special interest groups in this area of practice (what literature recommendations did they have?) and search for websites that provide updates of research.

Insights were gained from the literature and from consultations with other clinicians working in the field (expertise of others finger). An important issue was how to ensure that the proposed project would assist clients to better understand how they could manage their lives. The team had many ideas about this, ranging from theoretical principles (such as psychosocial approaches to managing pain) to how many PowerPoint slides should be used. To provide some expertise in what governed effective education, a lecturer who was an expert in persuasive messages used for selling/marketing purposes was consulted. In a presentation to the team, it was stressed that no more than five ideas should be conveyed and that repetition was important. Following the recommendation, literature regarding the Persuasive Delivery model was consulted (Malouf, 1990). The general recommendation was that there should be a focus on a "snappy" way to convey the messages which should be presented in a clear and concise manner.

Another educational principle the team identified was the importance of engaging clients in the delivery of the education session. This knowledge came in part from the literature (Catalano et al., 2009; Liddle et al., 2015) but was also influenced by their own experience as the existing program sometimes included previous clients' perspectives. This exchange with former clients was viewed positively by the team. The literature described how presenters who lived with a condition were more credible than a health professional as they were living proof of the possibility of living a satisfactory life. However, this approach was ultimately rejected because of the limited time frame. One further promising educational approach was the importance of consultation with previous clients to ensure that the plans for the session were relevant. Once again, there was limited time for planning and no funding to support the costs of bringing people together to consult (context and environment finger).

Despite the frustration of not being able to fully implement the advice provided by the research about well-founded educational principles that were likely to influence the impact of the revised program, the team was still committed to trialing a program. After considerable discussion, it was decided to use a lecture-style presentation with Power-Point slides to ensure that concepts that were difficult to grasp (e.g., acute vs persistent pain and central sensitization) were clearly explained. The information on the slides was to be short, simple, and repetitive, with everyday, easy-to-understand words. The principles that are known to underpin effective education were useful to begin thinking about how a teaching session could be conducted but ultimately modified to suit the circumstances. A formal approach to presenting information was taken rather than having a focus on engaging the group members. This was governed by limited resources and illustrates that research and/or theory may not be applicable in its entirety because the context does not support it.

The desire to revise the team's approach to client education involved gaining agreement by all team members. While the team had functioned together for several years, they did not necessarily work from a common understanding of pain management. One strategy used to bring about cohesion is to have a theoretical model that is shared by all team members. In pain management, it was recommended that this should be the biopsychosocial model (Gatchel & Howard, 2008). The team agreed to use this on the understanding that it would provide a common basis for the work the team was doing.

THE TRIAL SESSION

The team ran a four-hour education trial located at the hospital. The basic program was like the content and approach used in the existing eight-week program. Thus, despite understanding principles such as having previous clients come in to talk and engaging in learning exercises that would stimulate rethinking of current methods of managing pain, the pragmatic issues led to recycling existing procedures rather than a complete envisaging of the workshop techniques implemented.

From feedback at the end of the trial, it was evident that clients considered that consultation with the pain specialist was needed to kickstart any change of thinking regarding treatment options. The medical model was well entrenched in the clients' thinking and there was not a lot of conviction that a self-supportive model would be accepted prior to the consultation. While this was disappointing for the team, through reflection they identified what they had learned from the experience. For instance, the intentions of the project might not have matched the clients' expectations. As one team member noted, a shift in belief and behavior is needed which can be difficult to achieve in a very short time frame. The environment created in the revised approach encouraged "reflection" and "questioning," providing an opportunity for the client group to acquire information about each other's ways of managing pain. Understanding that there are different approaches to making changes was a positive outcome of the session. The team realized that focusing on a self-management approach rather than the shortening of the waiting list held great value and had potential for "snapshot" education sessions being used by the service in the future.

The process of trialing a revised program was a useful learning exercise as it became evident that there were several considerations (all linked to the context and environment finger). This included practical issues related to gaining people's engagement. For instance, transport, work, and family obligations made it difficult for some to attend and to travel into the city. Twenty people on the waiting list were invited but only five attended. From the team's perspective, booking a room at the hospital was a major task as there was limited availability. They also needed to find a time that suited all members of the pain team. There was no allocation of time to run this session – it stemmed from a genuine conviction that there was a better way to support their clients.

Finally, different issues were related to the team itself. For instance, one of the team members was resistant to the new venture yet persisted in being involved. The team members worked in a variety of wards in the hospital, which affected team cohesion, and they noted that having a dispersed team impacted on a sense of team collegiality and support for colleagues. Also, they realized that they misunderstood the triage process used at the hospital and were astonished by this.

In their reflections on the trial, the team members were surprised that many clients declined to attend the pilot education session. They were also disappointed that the feedback was not as positive and appreciative as they had expected. There was agreement that introducing a culture of self-management when people expect a "fix" is a big challenge. Clients' expectation was that they would be seen by a doctor in a clinic and they were suspicious that if they attended the education session, they would miss their appointment with the pain consultant. The team members learned that it took time for client expectations to change.

Despite the challenges in implementing this type of service delivery, the team considered that it was worth repeating and making use of their learning. One challenge was the difficulty of helping clients change beliefs about pain management in a short time frame. However, it was noted that the act of bringing people together in a workshop enabled them to question and challenge one another and learn that there are different responses to making lifestyle changes.

TIPS FOR USING RESEARCH AND LITERATURE

A list of tasks to inform the team about a revised program for persistent pain was described at the outset of this chapter but the reality was that a limited inquiry process was implemented. The team relied heavily on the expertise of individual team members, their general knowledge of other pain management programmes and the evidence they had accrued as individual clinicians that convinced them that a particular program would serve their purposes well. Of note, there were no reflections by any of the team on the potential of looking more carefully at the literature beyond the one study they had heard about at a conference. This could have been for several reasons, including the relationships between team members and overall dynamics of the team, or a lack of skills and resources to guide literature searching.

TYPES OF LITERATURE

There are many resources that can be used to provide information about a clinical question. Accessing research that has been published in credible journals is always a good option, but the expansion of EBP across sectors has led to an increasing variety of types of literature.

- **Articles that report on a specific research project**: research methods may include quantitative, qualitative, or mixed methods. It is important to read the research through the lens of how trustworthy it is and how relevant for your purposes.

- **Research summaries**: such as systematic reviews (and metaanalyses) and scoping reviews. A scoping review seeks to present an overview of a potentially large and diverse body of literature about a general topic. A systematic review is more specific and provides a detailed summary of the available research related to a research question. Search: "systematic review" or "scoping review" and your topic of interest.

- **Cochrane Library**: a collection of databases providing access to high-quality research evidence to inform healthcare decision making. It also includes the Cochrane Reviews, a database of systematic reviews and metaanalyses. Search: www.cochranelibrary.com, then browse by topic. It provides a summary of the available research within a stated time frame.

- **Critically Appraised Topics (CAT)**: provide summaries of research evidence as an answer to a developed clinical question. Practitioners value short summaries as these are quick to read and make sense of in a busy workplace (Robertson et al., 2013); CATs are an example of such summaries. They are available online for a variety of health professions.

- **Gray literature**: this includes theses, professional nonpeer-reviewed magazines, reports, working papers, government documents, and conference proceedings. They provide current information but may be geographically specific or culturally orientated and can be intended for small audiences. They may

be variable in quality and are not always "academic" but can provide a richer source of information than a scientific study.

- **Textbooks**: written by subject experts; may include theoretical arguments and research summaries as well as "what works," i.e., clinical expertise. This might also include discussions on Indigenous knowledge and insights into some of the ways in which knowledge is generated aside from Western scientific research strategies.

- **Artificial intelligence (AI)**: a recent development is the use of AI to search literature. This has been reported in medical literature as being a promising approach which will ultimately provide a speedy method of gathering relevant data (Schoeb et al., 2020).

See Grant and Booth (2009) for a typology of 14 review types.

CHECKING CREDIBILITY OF SOURCES

Guidelines are available to help you check the strength of the published research and its relevance to your practice. One example is McMaster's guidelines for critical appraisal of qualitative and quantitative studies, and systematic reviews, available online from McMaster University. Another is the CRAAP test (Blakeslee, 2004), a catchy acronym that can help to evaluate the credibility of a source (e.g., books, websites, journals). The acronym stands for:

- Currency: Is the source up to date?
- Relevance: Is the source relevant to your research?

- Authority: Where is the source published? Who is the author? Are they considered reputable and trustworthy in their field?
- Accuracy: Is the source supported by evidence? Are the claims cited correctly?
- Purpose: What was the motive behind publishing this source?

Websites may provide overviews of current evidence related to specialty practice areas. There is a plethora of websites and emerging issues related to research misrepresentation on websites that look plausible at first glance, and so checking the credibility of the website is important. There are numerous tools available to help with assessing website credibility, and research into what websites are most credible is emerging, hampered by the ever-changing nature of the internet (Bernstam et al., 2005). An example of a tool is www.easybib.com/ guides/citation-guides/citation- basics/how-to-tell-if-website-is- credible

There are many sources of evidence in the literature and many guidelines that may be used to critique the research that underpin the claims about the value of a particular intervention. See Atkinson and Cipriani (2018) for an overview of how to carry out a literature review.

Various frameworks are recommended for structuring a search. The PICO (Patient, Intervention, Comparison, Outcome) framework (Richardson et al., 1995) is commonly used but others exist that may be more appropriate for questions about health policy and management, such as ECLIPSE (Wildridge & Bell, 2002) (Expectation, Client Group, Location, Impact, Professionals, Service) or SPICE (Setting, Perspective, Intervention, Comparison, Evaluation) (Booth, 2006) for

service evaluation. However, before conducting a comprehensive literature search, an initial background search of the literature can provide valuable information as to how much literature for a given review question already exists and its general features/orientation. For instance, it may reveal whether systematic reviews have already been undertaken for a particular search question. Thus, the initial stage of the search for literature is to explore the situation you are interested in.

Once initial foraging has revealed if there is any literature related to your query as well as exposed you to questions that might arise from the studies already completed, then it is essential to draw from an extensive, organized search of the literature. The PICO framework is a useful structure for this; Jensen (2018) has helpfully developed a seven-step process to implementing the PICO framework.

Examples of two possible PICO questions for the pain management project are: For people suffering from persistent pain (P), how effective are active self-management strategies (I), compared to biomedical treatment approaches (C), in controlling pain (O)?

OR

For people with persistent pain who are waiting to see a consultant (P), would a pre-consultation workshop (I) enable them to manage their pain (O)? (NB: It is not always essential to have a comparative intervention.)

As can be seen, the two questions will lead to different literature searches. This exercise serves to clarify the aim of the study and thus the focus of the literature review. Once the essential research question is identified, then the various resources described above can be used as tools to critique the quality of the research.

In the pain management project, the team failed to start by developing a focused question.

REFLECTIONS OF THE TEAM ON THEIR PROJECT

This section provides an overview of the team's reflection on their project and their learning related to implementing this new service. It is summarized under the FFF with a focus on the use of literature.

Research and Literature

The team's reflection: the literature search had not been as extensive as we had intended. The temptation was to be solution focused and align ourselves with a particular study that appeared to be consistent with our intentions. We did not even look for a Cochrane Review. It was considered that chatting to the authors of a recent study would be sufficient. Time was an issue in this endeavor. We discussed how this might have been addressed. Perhaps the library staff could have assisted, or a student. The other issue was the skills and time needed to carry out an analysis of the research and make comparisons between studies. A senior student in any one of the professions might have assisted with this. Better collaborative links with the local university might have led to students assisting in the project.

Although it had been noted that there were several differences between the research context in the study and that of our trial, it was thought that we had taken account of these elements. However, there were more differences than we had paid attention to. We discovered that there were many questions that needed to be asked in the initial stages: what were clients' views on using a psychosocial approach; what were managers' expectations of the clinicians' roles; what educational approach would be most relevant? Each question has the potential to raise another question that could be answered by exploring literature, i.e., to understand the best way to develop an education program for the clients, an overview of many aspects was needed. Using someone else's program from another country was not necessarily the best solution for our specific environment.

Context and Environment

The team's reflection: eventually, it was realized that it was important to pay attention to the setting (the context and culture). This element was not spelled out in the research articles. In a literature review done in haste, the focus was on the techniques needed to implement a program with little consideration of the specific local context. Resources such as availability of rooms to run the sessions and staff time were critical in the project. Thus, the views of hospital managers needed to be ascertained – was the program an acceptable practice to them? It turned out that our proposed service was not supported by management, i.e., medical interventions were supported rather than self-management approaches.

On reflection, a business plan that spelt out cost benefits might have been helpful to make a case and win support. However, it was thought that this formal approach would have increased workloads and dulled enthusiasm. More questions needed to be asked of the research literature to ascertain if it would "work" in our environment. One of our key learnings was that despite the need to help clients shift their mindset from a passive medical model to an active biopsychosocial model of pain management, the medical model was reinforced by the system. Context is a significant aspect in the successful implementation of new services.

The Client

It is important to obtain clients' views on the intervention being considered. This information can be found from a range of sources. For instance, specific studies that report on clients' responses to being involved in a specific project might be found in sources of information such as websites, textbooks, and informal journals.

The team's reflection: while the original intention had been to discuss our ideas with past clients, this never occurred. As identified previously, some team members were surprised that clients might want this educational opportunity. However, it is known that clients are reluctant to give up on a "cure." Nevertheless, this fact was never really raised in our discussions, our orientation being to provide what we considered to be the best approach rather than ascertaining if clients thought it was a promising idea. Literature that addressed the question of what worked for the clients needed to be located. Addressing the experiences and concerns of the client group is particularly important in a program that is orientated toward helping people make behavioral changes.

Expertise of Others

Experts do not necessarily agree on what is "best practice." This information can be found by exploring the literature and making comparisons between the results of the studies. Finding out what is generally accepted, as well as where any differences lie, will encourage a critical review of the studies.

The team's reflection: there was considerable expertise within the team. We were committed to the idea of changing the focus of the program from a medical orientation to one of self-management. However, bringing our expertise to the situation was not enough. We also needed a questioning approach rather than expecting to find the ideal solution in the literature. Sharing knowledge between different team members was not seen as a priority. Having someone facilitate a session where the views of all team members were explored

might have given us a greater awareness of the different perspectives in the team.

Self

In this instance, the "self" refers both to the individuals in the team, and to the team due to the collective and collaborative nature of the reasoning for the team.

The team's reflection: the team became aware of a lack of opportunities to develop knowledge of how to search for literature as well as skills in debating issues related to client care. We met with a specific purpose of identifying how we might maintain a consistent attitude of enquiry. We came up with several strategies that encourage reviewing literature in ways that can become the norm. We planned to discuss these ideas with colleagues.

- Running a journal club to review current literature.
- Presenting reflections on practice, e.g., case reviews that include a focus on literature to support practice.
- Accessing in-service education on critiquing literature/research methods, e.g., from a librarian or a researcher.
- Ensuring feedback from conferences and training sessions is shared.
- Remaining motivated to stay alert for relevant literature, using the skills of a librarian or colleagues engaged in research.
- Making connections with educational institutions and requesting that students assist in locating, reviewing, and discussing literature.
- Setting up ongoing searches of literature with expectations of sharing findings on a regular basis; critical review of these with colleagues.
- Reviewing team processes and practices against best practice evidence regularly.

DISCUSSION

Most members of the group had read the research that emanated from the Australian research article. However, locating a breadth of relevant articles is the key task in any start-up study – the abstracts can be reviewed, and decisions made from reading those alone, only the relevant articles need be read in full. Typically, those involved in postgraduate education have the confidence to evaluate research while others who are primarily clinicians grow their knowledge through practice, reflection, and sharing ideas (Gabbay & le May, 2004). The team were all experienced clinicians not currently involved with postgraduate studies. Like all those who have completed postgraduate education, they had learned how to find and evaluate research and were aware of the importance of ensuring that practice is supported by credible research. There was, however, a strong opinion that contacting people who had developed successful programs to discuss their strategies was also an effective way to develop a program that would work. Explanations related to local practice could be readily obtained and questions asked to find out the nuts and bolts of how to set up an effective program. It was certainly helpful to have the article that summarized the research, but this was reviewed for its ideas about how to plan and implement a program rather than critiqued for the research standards. As noted in Gabbay and le May's (2004) study of mindlines, even if clinicians have the skills and interest in evaluating the literature, there is often minimal time allocated to developing new ideas and it will depend on clinician passion and a supportive team.

IMPLICATIONS FOR EDUCATION

Appropriate use of research literature has been the main support for best practice and has been widely promoted in educational programs for health professionals. This view of practice has been developed from a quantifiable perspective of evidence and was largely influenced by Cochrane's conclusion that research based on randomized trials "offer(s) the most unbiased way of determining whether a treatment works" (Spring et al., 2019, p. 10). Ultimately, the Cochrane Collaboration was developed to provide a central system of trials that can be used with confidence by clinicians and policy makers to provide reliable evidence for practice. However, a further issue that was subsequently raised by a group from McMaster's University was the observation that clinicians rarely used this type of "best evidence" when making clinical decisions about patient care. Instead, treatment decisions were thought to be more often influenced by several factors such as personal experience when training and during practice, the practitioner's capacity for and habits in critical reflection (Benfield & Jeffery, 2022), interaction with colleagues, and an over-riding concern about liability (Spring et al., 2019).

This refocusing of what constitutes evidence from the more formal research results located in the literature to strategies that make use of the views of experienced practitioners and clients has been referred to as "two cliffs," i.e., the scientific evidence cliff and the patient/practitioner cliff (Aas & Alexanderson, 2012). The more tangible sources such as research literature (the scientific cliff) can be readily understood as providing evidence that is "reliable" but does have the added complexity of needing to fully understand the research methods and to critique the findings in relation to a specific clinical situation. This is a challenge for students and novice practitioners who have limited knowledge of research, but it is also difficult for practitioners who may have restricted research knowledge and very little time to find the resources and critically evaluate them. The less tangible sources of evidence arising from practitioner/client interaction is an important focus in practice where determination of the client's needs is seen as pivotal (the patient/practitioner "cliff"). Although being integral to practice, it is not readily discussed explicitly. There is even less analysis of how EBP is taught and then transferred to practice (i.e., the "bridge"). Lecturer ideals may not be consistent with practitioners' realities, leading to students getting mixed messages about what constitutes effective evidence-based strategies.

For the development of a profession, it is essential that novice therapists can take a critical view of practice decisions. Commonly, EBP is mainly seen to be solely related to searching for and critiquing literature to provide a credible underpinning for practice. There are many reasons why EBP is not as simple as learning and applying a set of skills related to evaluating research. This theoretical information needs to be integrated into decision making that also takes account of contextual issues such as the client's circumstances, their needs and opinions, the practitioner's knowledge, the workplace culture, and the resources available (Craik & Rappolt, 2003). Of note, the most difficult aspect is the integration of evidence for actual decision making (Thomas et al., 2012). Additionally, there may be little or no evidence available in the research literature and in particular, evidence related to cultural variations in health (Pitima et al., 2017). It may be equally important to use a range of alternative sources such as practitioner networks, clients' stories, workplace protocols, workshop information, and other condensed summaries to find the best basis for decision making within a realistic time frame (Robertson et al., 2013).

This chapter identifies the complexity of ensuring that practice is based on evidence. The format of the FFF provides a way of thinking laterally about the components

that determine best practice. It is important that education programs teach in ways that highlight the diversity of practice, including the environmental components that affect the implementation of research findings. This involves using real problems of practice. For example, while students are on placement, they ask critical questions about the supporting evidence retrospectively once they have understood the issues; or while on campus the tasks given to develop analytical skills are directly related to the real world of practice where context matters. Using real scenarios provided by current clinicians and returned to them for comment is another strategy (Scott et al., 2011).

Finally, the use of narratives such as those used in this book is a teaching method that stimulates the linking of learning with prior experience by engaging emotions. Stories show "learners how they are positioned within and shaped by larger cultural narratives" (Clark & Rossiter, 2008, p. 6). These authors recommend the use of autobiographical learning portfolios. The FFF provides a valuable tool by identifying a range of elements that could be included in such stories about decision making.

CONCLUSION

In this instance, there was no perceived need to search further than the program the team had heard about from the conference and reading the related article. The biggest issue at the outset was the team's desire to decrease client time on the waiting list. In essence, they took a pragmatic approach – if a program worked for their Australian colleagues, that was good enough as an indication of its likely success. In fact, they were excited about the prospect of duplicating this study. Motivating clinicians to go beyond their usual responsibilities and understanding is critical to the success of new ideas.

As illustrated by the scenario in this chapter, enthusiasm is not enough. Searching the literature is rather like a journey where one road leads to another. Ideally, it is important to explore the situation and go to the literature with several ideas/ questions to test. Only then is it possible to search the literature extensively and strategically to find well-conceived studies that have similar features to the context of those wishing to implement new ideas. The complexity of formally checking out the published research can deter practitioners from doing this. Time limitations in practice are an important consideration. As suggested earlier, ascertaining credibility of the research could be an effective use of time. Additionally, using literature that provides a critical summary of research studies such as systematic reviews and the Cochrane collection can provide a synopsis of the strength of evidence.

The team learned that faithful replication of specific research is often not possible. There are invariably contextual issues that impact on the success of a program. As already noted, aspects such as availability of rooms were an issue which seemed small in the scheme of things but were frustrating. A bigger issue in the project was the discovery about how entrenched clients were in a medical focus on their issues whereas the team viewed the psychosocial approach as the way forward as these were people for whom there was no known "medical" intervention. Consistent with social constructivist theory, searching for understanding is a process where professionals use past experiences and their own "know-how" to create personal meaning (Thomas et al., 2014). They are therefore active problem solvers and constructors of their own knowledge. While the literature exploration in this scenario might not have been of the highest order, the team members have enhanced their understanding of both what is essential in carrying out a well-thought-through literature search and what constitutes an effective client education program (Figure 7.1, Table 7.1).

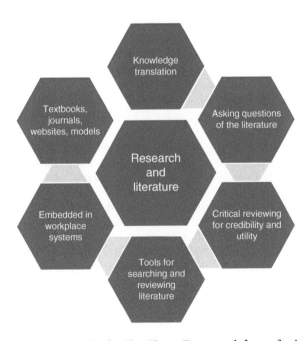

FIGURE 7.1   Research and literature in the Five Finger Framework for professional reasoning.

TABLE 7.1   Key Points

Role	Key Points
Practitioner/student	• Consult with colleagues as you generate the relevant question prior to literature search. • Understand how to access and use databases available to you. • Do a two-stage literature exploration process. Tease out the questions that you have regarding the topic of choice, then do a well-focused search using a tool such as PICO. • Search for well-synthesized general documents first, e.g., national/government/World Health Organization clinical guidelines. • Include systematic reviews or critically appraised topics in search terms. • Use a specific tool to critique the research literature you have selected, e.g., ECPLISE, SPICE. • Read research literature for utility – what's the fit with your context? • Appreciate the need for contextualization of research evidence. • Make a habit of reading journal articles; keep a reading log – even one article a month once you have graduated will help you maintain a focus on the research evidence. • Use the FFF template for decisions and ensure key references are included.

Educator	• Use the FFF to generate questions and information prior to any literature review.
	• Scaffold use of literature in class and assignment writing.
	  1. Provide all references for students to read and include in assignment.
	  2. Provide key references and request that students find an additional two or three.
	  3. Increase the expectation that they find literature gradually; always provide key or seminal readings.
	• Teach the use of specific tools for literature searching and critiquing.
	• Encourage use of research reviews that are well synthesized and trustworthy.
	• Provide list of recommended websites; students may not have the knowledge required to adequately assess trustworthiness of websites.
	• Learn about AI and how it can be safely used.
	• Use case study research to nurture understanding of the client.
	• Have students keep a reading log and nurture habits of reading that will be realistic in practice.
	• Link fieldwork education experiences to research and literature.
	  1. Reflection on a client and find key literature that justifies what they saw/did in practice.
	  2. Reflection on a client and find literature that informs what alternative research-based techniques or approaches could have been used.
	  3. Reflection on the service and find key government-level policy and direction that influence the service.
	• Teach effective use of librarian services.

TABLE 7.1   (Continued)

Role	Key Points
Manager	• Ensure access to essential current literature. • Establish processes that ensure protocols and guidelines are research evidence based and updated regularly. • Provide easy pathways that practitioners can use to present their research ideas. • Ensure that there are ways for clinicians to continue to learn how to search for and critique the literature effectively (e.g., workshops, ongoing in-services). • Create an expectation that research is used and justified in case presentations, new intervention strategies, etc. • Cultivate a culture of enquiry. • Support academic discourse in the workplace, e.g., journal club, research evidence folder. • Support a process for knowledge translation, e.g., experienced practitioners guide intervention plans and check against research evidence. • Minimize the need for individuals to search and synthesis literature; have processes that ensure research-based evidence is embedded in the service. • Use librarian services. • Support questioning of practice so that questioning literature is triggered when necessary. • Have up-to-date textbooks in the workplace. • Form and nurture relationships with academic environment. • Ensure feedback from conferences and training is shared with teams. • Have students on fieldwork education with you share research evidence.
Supervisor	• Use the FFF to assist practitioners to check out their ideas and justify decisions with a focus on the research and literature. • Help the supervisee contextualize research findings. • Make links with the supervisee between what they are experiencing and research-based evidence. • Cultivate and nurture curiosity about knowledge that sits behind practice. • Keep supervisees' level of experience and knowledge front of mind; minimize expectations on novices for complex and time-consuming knowledge translation.

This is the final chapter in relation to the five fingers on the framework. The tools provided in Chapter 9 include techniques for integrating research and literature into reasoning using the FFF. The next chapter delves into transdisciplinarity, exploring the cross-over of knowledges and practices between disciplines.

REFERENCES

Aas, R. W., & Alexanderson, K. (2012). Challenging evidence-based decision-making: a hypothetical case study about return to work. *Occupational Therapy International*, *19*(1), 28–44.

Atkinson, L. Z., & Cipriani, A. (2018). How to carry out a literature search for a systematic review: a practical guide. *BJPsych Advances*, *24*(2), 74–82.

Benfield, A., & Jeffery, H. (2022). Exploring evidence based practice implementation by occupational therapists: implications for fieldwork. *Journal of Occupational Therapy Education*, *6*(4), 10.

Bernstam, E. V., Shelton, D. M., Walji, M., & Meric-Bernstam, F. (2005). Instruments to assess the quality of health information on the world wide web: what can our patients actually use? *International Journal of Medical Informatics*, *74*(1), 13–19.

Blakeslee, S. (2004). The CRAAP test. *LOEX Quarterly*, *31*(3), 4.

Booth, A. (2006). Clear and present questions: formulating questions for evidence-based practice. *Library Hi Tech*, *24*(3)), 355–368.

Catalano, T., Kendall, E., Vandenberg, A., & Hunter, B. (2009). The experiences of leaders of self-management courses in Queensland: exploring health professional and peer leaders' perceptions of working together. *Health & Social Care in the Community*, *17*(2), 105–115.

Clark, M. C., & Rossiter, M. (2008). Narrative learning in adulthood. *New Directions for Adult and Continuing Education*, *2008*(119), 61–70.

Craik, J., & Rappolt, S. (2003). Theory of research utilization enhancement: a model for occupational therapy. *Canadian Journal of Occupational Therapy*, *5*, 266–275.

Davies, S., Quintner, J., Parsons, R., Parkitny, L., Knight, P., Forrester, E., Roberts, M., Graham, C., Visser, E., Antill, T., Packer, T., &

Schug, S. (2011a). Preclinic group education sessions reduce waiting times and costs at public pain medicine units. *Pain Medicine*, *12*(1), 59–71.

Davies, S. J., Hayes, C., & Quintner, J. L. (2011b). System plasticity and integrated care: Informed consumers guide clinical reorientation and system reorganization. *Pain Medicine*, *12*(1), 4–8.

Gabbay, J., & le May, A. (2004). Evidence based guidelines or collectively constructed "mindlines?" Ethnographic study of knowledge management in primary care. *British Medical Journal (Clinical Research)*, *329*(7473), 1013.

Gatchel, R., & Howard, K. (2008). The biopsychosocial approach. *Practical Pain Management*, *8*(4). www.practicalpain-management.com/treatments/psycho-logical/biopsychosocial-approach

Grant, M. J., & Booth, A. (2009). A typology of reviews: an analysis of 14 review types and associated methodologies. *Health Information & Libraries Journal*, *26*(2), 91–108.

Jensen, K.A. (2018). 7 Steps to the Perfect Pico Search. Evidence-Based Nursing Practice. www.ebsco.com/sites/g/files/nabnos191/files/acquiadam-assets/7-Steps-to-the-Perfect-PICO-Search-White-Paper_0.pdf

Liddle, J., Liu, X., Aplin, T., & Gustafsson, L. (2015). The experiences of peer leaders in a driving cessation programme. *British Journal of Occupational Therapy*, *78*(6), 383–390.

Malouf, D. (1990). *How to create and deliver a dynamic presentation*. Simon & Schuster.

Pitama, S. G., Bennett, S. T., Waikaremoana Waitoki, T. N., Haitana, H. V., Pahina, J., Taylor, J. E., Tassell-Matamua, N., Lutz Beckert, L. R., Palmer, S. C., Huria, T. M., Lacey, C. J., & McLachlan, A. (2017). A proposed hauora Māori clinical guide for psychologists: using the hui process and Meihana model in clinical assessment and formulation. *New Zealand Journal of Psychology*, *46*(3), 7–19.

Richardson, W. S., Wilson, M. C., Nishikawa, J., & Hayward, R. S. (1995). The well-built clinical question: a key to evidence-based decisions. *ACP Journal Club*, *123*(3), A12–A13.

Robertson, L., Graham, F., & Anderson, J. (2013). What actually informs practice: occupational therapists' views of evidence. *British Journal of Occupational Therapy*, *76*(7), 317–324.

Schoeb, D., Suarez-Ibarrola, R., Hein, S., Dressler, F. F., Adams, F., Schlager, D., & Miernik, A. (2020). Use of artificial intelligence for medical literature search: randomized controlled trial using the Hackathon format. *Interactive Journal of Medical Research*, *9*(1), e16606.

Scott, P. J., Altenburger, P. A., & Kean, J. (2011). A collaborative teaching strategy for enhancing learning of evidence-based clinical decision-making. *Journal of Allied Health*, *40*(3), 120–127.

Spring, B., Marchese, S. H., & Steglitz, J. (2019). History and process of evidence-based practice in mental health. In S. Dimidjian (Ed.), *Evidence-based practice in action: Bridging clinical science and intervention* (pp. 9–27). Guilford Press.

Thomas, A., Menon, A., Boruff, J., Rodriguez, A. M., & Ahmed, S. (2014). Applications of social constructivist learning theories in knowledge translation for healthcare professionals: a scoping review. *Implementation Science*, *9*(1), 54.

Thomas, A., Saroyan, A., & Snider, L. M. (2012). Evidence-based practice behaviours: a comparison amongst occupational therapy students and clinicians. *Canadian Journal of Occupational Therapy*, *79*(2), 96–107.

Watson, E., Cosio, D., & Lin, E. (2014). Mixed-method approach to veteran satisfaction with pain education. *Journal of Rehabilitation Research and Development*, *51*, 503–514.

Wildridge, V., & Bell, L. (2002). How CLIP became ECLIPSE: a mnemonic to assist in searching for health policy/management information. *Health Information and Libraries Journal*, *19*(2), 113–115.

CHAPTER 8

Synthesizing World Views

Transdisciplinarity and the Five Finger Framework

Jan Hendrik Roodt
Advanced Academic Facilitator, Te Pūkenga, New Zealand

INTRODUCTION

The wisdom that health practitioners draw on every day includes a wide range of disciplines and world views. Occupational therapy is one such profession where one of the key approaches is pragmatic problem solving. Like some of the other multidisciplinary vocations, including system design engineering, information technology practitioners, and those in multi-resource agriculture, the question of who we are and what we do is not easy to answer. Nor is it easy to manage the uncertainty and risks inherent in practicing within a field with such a broad scope.

This chapter covers the concept of transdisciplinarity working within, across, and beyond the traditional disciplines, as a way of explaining what practitioners do, how they do it, and how they make decisions under uncertainty. We use the profession of occupational therapy to illustrate some points, but this chapter is neither solely about

nor for occupational therapists. The ethical imperative is included in the discussion as a moral position, a "Values North Star". It opens a way of acting and doing in a manner that potentially grounds work in a deeper respectful, responsible foundation, and points to shifts in how one approaches the education of future practitioners.

CONTEXT

I would like to share this story so that readers can see that the problem is not the need for help; the problem is what people do to help – when it is aligned with the absolute belief that what one is doing is the only solution (Grootjans, 2010, p. 225).

Reflecting on his work as a European (western paradigm) health practitioner in the Northern Territory of Australia, Grootjans

Professional Reasoning in Healthcare: Navigating Uncertainty Using the Five Finger Framework, First Edition.
Edited by Helen Jeffery, Linda Robertson, Jan Hendrik Roodt, and Susan Ryan.
© 2024 John Wiley & Sons Ltd. Published 2024 by John Wiley & Sons Ltd.

tells the story of getting to grips with Aboriginal culture. His western knowledge and ways of doing clash with the world view of those he hopes to help. He concludes that one's enthusiastic efforts can often lead to more harm than good, and particularly in dimensions of society that one does not consider to be influenced by the interventions. The spiritual expression of ethnic groups, for example, that of the San in the southern regions of Africa, is a good example. It is now believed that the San (a broad collective of First Nations people) were part of the first anatomically human beings and that their spiritual worldviews may be as old as 30 000 years. The Khoe-Sān of the Kalahari are known for ritual dance for individual and social healing and bonding (Afolayan, 2004). Preserving this legacy is a high priority for the South African government but it raises the question: are the efforts by well-meaning workers inadvertently locking the San into a position that might make it impossible for them to adjust to the world as it advances? How will this impact the San as a people (Lewis-Williams & Pearce, 2004)?

Current practice in occupational therapy and other broad fields like information and communication technology, and systems engineering is deeply rooted in western science and philosophy. The western world view and education hold a dominant position, often considering as relevant only the knowledge generated from within this philosophical paradigm. Indigenous peoples view the world through their own philosophical lens. They have their own systems of logic and discourse. In New Zealand, the Māori world view is "informed by collective and intergenerational wisdom" (Ruwhiu & Cathro, 2014, p. 4). The position is that there are underlying epistemological assumptions to sense making that are specific to Kaupapa Māori, or the Māori way, and this is different from a western epistemology.

Iwama et al. (2009) introduced the Kawa model as a culturally responsive alternative model to western approaches for Japanese occupational therapists. Using the metaphor of a river that meanders through a landscape, it considers "the life path of a client, be it person, group or organisation" (MacLeod Schroeder, 2018, p. 39). The client is part of a dynamic landscape that interacts in many ways from outside and within.

Hammell and Iwama (2012) raise the issue of the human right to wellbeing and ask if there is too much of a focus by occupational therapists on dysfunction. Should more attention be paid to interventions that support meaningful occupation that contribute to the individual and communal wellbeing? They argue that striving to change the dynamics and dimensions of "physical, cultural, social, political, legal, or economic environment to counter discrimination and to equalize opportunities . . . is a political act" (p. 390). Such a broad transgressive stance may not be within the sphere of influence of individual practitioners, but it does hint at an ethical imperative that will be discussed later in this chapter.

The experience of Grootjans is a signpost; for occupational therapy, one could state that putting the wellbeing of the client front and center of the work means taking into account a much broader view of the world in which we practice. The next section examines recent developments in knowledge generation and dealing with complex situations that may cross cultural and other boundaries. Finally, strategies are introduced based on the transdisciplinarity concept to support the artful practice of occupational therapy within a transdisciplinary value system.

TRANSDISCIPLINARITY: ORIGINS, PHILOSOPHY, AND PRACTICE

Transdisciplinarity is a recent approach to generating understanding and knowledge. It was formally introduced by Jean Piaget in 1970 at a conference where the narrow nature of disciplinary education at universities was being discussed (Nicolescu, 2006). It is worth unpacking the word "transdisciplinary" because when Piaget used it, he was careful not to upset his audience. He spoke in vague terms of a super level of working amongst disciplines, something without boundaries. Nicolescu is of the opinion that Piaget purposefully focused only on the meaning "across" and "between" that the Latin prefix "trans" signifies. At the same conference, the Austrian Erich Jantsch defined transdisciplinarity as a hyperdiscipline. A hyperdiscipline is situated as a super coordinator between the disciplines of the teaching system and derives innovation based on an axiomatic approach. Axioms are statements that are self-evident or intuitively true and serve as the foundation of a theory.

A hyperdiscipline is not what Piaget had in mind, according to Nicolescu. He is quick to give credit to Jantsch for the idea of an axiomatic basis for transdisciplinarity, while insisting that Piaget intended the prefix "trans" also to mean "beyond." In the field of health practice, some state that transdisciplinarity aims to holistically integrate disciplinary knowledge, transcending traditional boundaries, asking practitioners to work collaboratively with others to address common problems (Choi & Pak, 2006; Fitzmaurice & Richmond, 2017). On the other hand, fusion across disciplines is not transdisciplinarity, but links and bridges are feasible and make possible the migration of ideas from one discipline to another (Nicolescu, 2014).

Despite the perceived value of transdisciplinary therapy models, it was reported by Young (2019) that in school settings, client therapy services are often limited to consultation and collaboration. The problem is that in the consultative approach, there is a limited degree of involvement by the client in bringing their world view to bear on the proposed intervention. In a participatory approach, all the actors are equally responsible for the derived intervention (Mobjörk, 2010): the healthcare practitioner, the client, and all relevant stakeholders, including family and cultural advisors in many cases.

Action in society and practice are seldom organized along the lines of the modern disciplines as presented at universities (Montuori & Donnelly, 2016). The transdisciplinary movement also responded to the need to address complex societal issues (Neuhauser, 2018), which is hampered by the limited interaction between the professional practitioner, policymakers, clients, and other stakeholders. Efforts fail when the individuals and teams have different views about what transdisciplinarity entails. Satterfield et al. (2009) reported that true transdisciplinary approaches would require shared goals based on client values, trust, leadership, and organizational structure. Roux et al. (2017), working on projects for ecological systems change, noted that transdisciplinarity within a practice setting can lead to mutual learning and new understanding by all the participants. It does this by challenging the concept of an expert who generates knowledge and transfers it to users. In fact, the benefits accrue when the perceived superiority of hard scientific data is addressed and all available knowledge, including informal and experiential knowledge, is treated on equal footing.

Transdisciplinarity is a formal theory and a way of practice, founded on a rigorous axiomatic basis. It argues for the existence and growth of disciplinary knowledge and practice, because without disciplines there is no trans-disciplinarity. From that position, based for example in evidence from modern physics and mathematics, it is described to mean between, across, and beyond the disciplines.

What sets true transdisciplinary thinking and doing apart from inter- and multidisciplinary approaches is the fundamental shift from seeing the world as a unit made up of intricately linked but separate parts supported by a knowable, testable, and predictable reality. Rather, the argument is that realities are constructed through experiences of what is *real* (the universal Reality which we as humanity cannot fathom), and knowledge and understanding are created as a collective effort in and between the minds of people (Stacey, 2001). There is a difference between what is *Real*, that which *is*, independent of what one perceives, and *reality*, that which is *plastic and changing* based on thoughts and actions (Cilliers & Nicolescu, 2012). Universal *Reality* has many dimensions or levels that are irreducible. It cannot be simplified.

The dimensions or levels/layers coexist and interact in many ways. Passing from one level of reality to a different one is experienced as a breakdown of fundamental concepts such as causality and when the laws of the system change. The very structure of reality, the constituent structural levels, is discontinuous. The levels do not form hierarchies and they can coexist and interact. A specific level of reality is what it is because all other levels exist at the same time. A given level of reality is thus governed by only a part of the totality of laws governing all levels, making that level *incomplete*. The incompleteness of levels is mathematically posited by Gödel's Incompleteness Theorem (Nagel & Newman, 2001).

What are the practical implications of this view of Reality? The fact that it is plastic and dynamic, based on the thoughts and actions of the observer, implies that there are related but different perspectives of reality. This is not to say that all things are "relative." Quite the opposite: by careful consideration, the difference and similarity can be evaluated and judged to understand different dimensions of reality. The possibility of coexistence of these levels of reality can be considered for the coherence of understanding. It is not only about the differences, but also about aspects that are similar that can be used to gain a deeper understanding. There is no complete set of governing laws for a set of realities, which means that one has the ability and opportunity to discover more governing principles. "When our perspectives of the world change, the world changes" (Nicolescu, 2010, p. 26). Human phenomena are not as predictable as those in nature and as such the description and understanding of any phenomenon can benefit from as many perspectives as possible.

An understanding of the different levels of reality can be negotiated by choosing an appropriate logic for reasoning. If there is agreement that there may be another level of reality (a third level when considering two contradictory realities), where what appears disunited or incongruent is in fact united and where a contradiction is lifted, the opposing views are resolved. It means being open to and actively working toward a new understanding – a new reality. One can bridge initial differences and come to a position that is of mutual benefit. An interesting example can be found in resource plundering: consider the killing of rhinos for their horns, used for ritual and medicinal purposes in some cultures. One position, or reality, is that rhinos are to be protected as an endangered species. The other position is that the rhino horn is a resource to be used by communities for financial income as it has perceived value as a medicine. By considering a logical position that rhinos need to be protected and that communities under financial pressure may need alternatives for income, a new reality of eco-tourism may be cocreated to achieve both goals. The third reality of rhino horn being perceived as having health benefits is harder to address, and may be shifted by the fact that the community poaching rhino horns are taken out of the supply chain, thus making trade in horns unsustainable (Koen et al., 2017).

If *Reality* is discontinuous, it can be postulated that there is a zone between levels and beyond all levels that is transparent to human experiences, descriptions, and formalisms. One cannot fathom this Hidden Third, or zone of nonresistance, as Nicolescu calls it. This Hidden Third corresponds to "the sacred." It is the source of transdisciplinary moral values. From this position, the practitioner is required to know the practice world. Being immersed in the Hidden Third, the practitioner, the client, and other stakeholders are interrelated. Nicolescu states that from a transdisciplinary viewpoint, complexity as described by philosophers like Morin (2008) and Cilliers (1998) is the modern understanding of the ancient concept of universal interdependence (Nicolescu, 2010, p. 31).

Many of the everyday problems faced in practice can be attended to easily. However, some problems include culture, technology, nature, and societal issues and they often involve several levels of reality. If one demands that only one reality exists, contradictory positions will quite likely emerge. This "preferred" reality would silence the other voices and insist on finding solutions that ignore the contradictions. Elevating a specific reality or giving it preference has the effect of neglecting the Hidden Third between that reality and others. Technology, for example, exists in the transdisciplinary zone of inanimate objects, but culture and society span the client and stakeholder spaces, the professional practitioner reality, and the Hidden Third. We intuitively know that in trying to unravel complex issues, we tend to discover even more questions. It is like tugging on a ball of string!

When engaging with a complex societal dilemma, choices are made about the description of the problem. Some aspects may receive more attention than others,

depending on how one judges the situation. For example, in a cultural or religious context where family members or societal leaders may hold positions of influence, this may shift the way in which the situation is evaluated and judged. These views, or mental models, are never complete which means, as was said before, that one cannot know these phenomena in a way that will allow one to determine how they will behave or unfold precisely over time. Practitioners are forced into an interpretation of the issues at hand and to evaluate things based on choices that cannot ultimately be justified in a fully objective fashion. As Woermann and Cilliers (2012) say, "Our modelling choices are based on subjective judgements about what matters – both in terms of our work and in terms of our personal lives" (p. 448). One recognizes, as a moral position, that all knowledge is limited because mental models are truncated and reduced versions of the world, anchored in time and space. Woermann and Cilliers (2012, p. 453) state that "a complex understanding of ethics posits the good as something which is necessarily subject to revision and deconstruction; and, hence as something which is provisional." Such an ethical "North Star" supports the artful practitioner to remain humble and critically reflexive.

IDENTITY AND A TRANSDISCIPLINARY VALUE SYSTEM

Occupational or professional identity is shaped by our ways of doing work, our ways of thinking about and making sense of ourselves, our relationship with others, and the relationship with the world we live in (Unruh, 2004; Whyte, 2009). These relationships are interwoven and influence each other (MacLeod Schroeder, 2018). As with systems engineering and information technology professionals, occupational therapists work in a field that covers overlapping disciplines. Not surprisingly, it is hard to describe these professions and as a result practitioners find it difficult to develop a professional work identity (Emes et al., 2005). Identity is reflected in the way in which one engages with practice and impacts our continuous learning in a transdisciplinary context (Nicolescu, 2018). This may occur through the following pathways.

- **Learning to know**: this includes education in the methods which help one separate the illusionary from the real and to have access to the extensive knowledge of our time. The *scientific spirit* is indispensable, and the goal is not to absorb and master the vast mass of knowledge. Constant questioning and debating of the facts, the patterns and formalizations are core tenets of this approach, while simultaneously building bridges between disciplines and practitioners.
- **Learning to do**: this is the development of the mastery of professional practice and agility in occupation. What is required is an "authentically woven occupation . . . bind(ing) together in the interior of human beings threads linking them to other occupations" (Nicolescu, 2018, p. 76), thus hinting at the concept of transferable skills.
- **Learning to make**: the doing of creative things, uncovering novel approaches, and innovative shifts of application are part of action and making a difference.
- **Learning to live together**: to go beyond tolerance of difference in the broadest and narrowest sense, including race, beliefs, and opinion.

From a transdisciplinary perspective, it highlights the need to always search for the AND rather than the OR in positions, finding the realities of coexistence, open to other world views.

- **Learning to be**: the ongoing apprenticeship and generating of knowledge in engagement beyond the disciplines of the field.

In practice, one should consider how to transcend the "common good" and work toward outcomes that are rich in opportunity for crafting responsible, acceptable, and defendable results. Which brings one to the concept of a moral ethical imperative mentioned earlier.

Woermann (2013) talks about virtues for a complex world and discusses three moral imperatives: *transgressivity*, *irony*, and *imagination*. These are not classic rules or yardsticks but tools suited to a complex world. These "tools" are products of how one frames the complex world. There is uncertainty and risk, and a moral duty to follow guiding principles when making choices and taking action. Knowledge claims are subject to being overturned and all claims are made within a certain context of realities. This concept of "provisionality" is important and hints at the dynamic nature of knowledge and approaches, urging one to practice in a humble manner.

- **Transgressivity**: one must accept the moral obligation to stay open to the unfolding of the world into an unpredictable future, while agreeing to respond innovatively to the issues being faced. This must happen with urgency and with action. In the process, boundaries and accepted views must be challenged. This should be done in a modest manner: first, one should challenge one's own position in the face of the possibility of other equally valid realities. Second, modesty is called for in the face of uncertainty, being aware of the open-ended nature of knowledge.

- **Irony**: this can best be described as the mismatch between what is expected based on the literal meaning of words and what is implied. In the case of transdisciplinarity, it can be interpreted as a need for improvising to deal with contradiction. One accepts that the unfolding realities are resulting from decisions. Decisions and actions may have unintended consequences (universal interdependence in complex systems). There is no final truth or final, ultimate, solution, only more suitable ones or less appropriate ones. It is ironic that we use our partial knowledge and limited personal experiences to question the world. Simply put, we should not take ourselves or our ideas too seriously as this would get in the way of acting responsibly in the face of complexity (Woermann, 2013).

- **Imagination**: to consider possibilities and to construct rich tapestries of outcomes, imagination is needed to explore other forms of wisdom. It aids the development of mental models in anticipation of outcomes based on actions that others, and we, may take. It requires a deep understanding of the perspectives of a range of stakeholders and how they are networked. This allows practitioners to plan critically for the future. The future will unfold in surprising ways, which means that uncertainty is part of the deal. How the professional practitioner responds with critical judgment to this uncertainty is

the moral imperative. There is also the tension between the imagined futures from contradictory perspectives/realities. Moral imagination supports recognition and integration of these viewpoints into realistic future solution spaces.

THE FIVE FINGER FRAMEWORK AND TRANSDISCIPLINARY PRACTICE

In the previous chapters, the metaphorical role of each finger was considered in some detail. The thumb represents the "self." The "self" has an identity that is evolving and changing through ongoing learning as described above by Nicolescu. The thumb interacts with the other four fingers in an iterative way to devise and deliver evidence-based interventions. The space for the intervention development and delivery process is structured around different subjective realities.

In the transdisciplinary paradigm, the evolving practitioner (the "self") is an intricate part of the changing community, client space, and environment. Every time the thumb touches the index finger, insight may be created or updated for the practitioner and the community of practitioners. When the thumb interacts with the middle finger – the client (as individual and collective) – both entities experience change and new learning. Conceivably, the thumb can touch both the index and middle fingers simultaneously in a group session. This process changes perception and interpretation of experiential knowledge. The changes and shifts are a result of the interrelated nature of all complex systems. Without oversimplifying, every interaction of the self with any other finger changes the identity of the hand and the intervention in the palm of that hand. That in turn impacts the field of practice.

Arguably, some of these changes are small and incremental, but inevitably they are unique, as every client is different and so is every practitioner. In terms of the levels of reality, one can see how the actions of the fingers are generative to construct new and shared realities. Returning to the Kawa model and the metaphor of the flowing river, what is imagined here is the confluence of several streams into a larger river. This new flow may diminish the effects of some objects washed in from upstream, while some effects may combine in unexpected ways to become significant characteristics of the new river. For example, a practitioner may consider a new client case and have an intuitive idea or hunch about possible courses of action. It may be confirmed during the first client facing meeting. However, after discussion of the case with a mentor or manager, some obstacles are raised in terms of regulatory changes perhaps. Or the client may challenge the practitioner world view.

As was argued for before, the Five Finger Framework (FFF) supports reflexive practice, learning, and sense making while fostering anticipatory thinking. When using other metaphors like the Kawa model, the FFF keeps the practitioner grounded in the interactive development and emerging interventions. A transdisciplinary way of thinking considers that there may be a range of different subjective realities at play, including those based on culture, religion, social standing, dogmatic principles, and different epistemologies. The practitioner must engage with knowledge and insight supported by context-specific world views. Judicious application of a provisional mindset under an ethical imperative ensures foregrounding of the physical, cultural, social, political, legal, and economic environments to counter discrimination and equalize opportunities.

CONCLUDING REMARKS

In a transdisciplinary paradigm (Figure 8.1), one must face multiple, constantly changing realities, recognizing the deeply connected

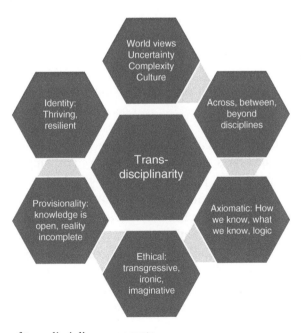

FIGURE 8.1   Overview of transdisciplinary concepts.

nature of the physical world and experiences. The approach expands the solution space by facilitating knowledge sharing and solution development by a broader stakeholder set, rather than focusing on the requirements and know-how of the initial owner of the problem and their reality. Seemingly contradictory perspectives may present themselves to a practitioner and in the process of collective sense making between the practitioner and other role players, new knowledge may be created. This process and the insights produced will vary from case to case and will be complex and constantly emerging in different, often unpredictable ways as the situation changes (McGregor, 2020).

A transdisciplinary position acknowledges the incompleteness of knowledge (it is forever under construction) and the provisionality of all claims and decisions. By integrating an ethical position, based on complexity theory, the principles of transdisciplinarity can be incorporated into the practice identity of practitioners. Building on a broad understanding of professional identity, this identity can be developed to be more resilient and to thrive. The FFF fits squarely into this developmental pathway as it fosters confident, respectful, and responsible reflective practice.

REFERENCES

Afolayan, F. S. (2004). *Culture and customs of South Africa*. Greenwood Press.

Choi, B. C. K., & Pak, A. W. P. (2006). Multidisciplinarity, interdisciplinarity and transdisciplinarity in health research, services, education and policy: 1. Definitions, objectives, and evidence of effectiveness. *Clinical and Investigative Medicine*, *29*(6), 351–364.

Cilliers, P. (1998). *Complexity and postmodernism – Understanding complex systems*. Routledge.

Cilliers, P., & Nicolescu, B. (2012). Complexity and transdisciplinarity – discontinuity, levels of reality and the hidden third. *Futures*, *44*(8), 711–718.

Emes, M., Smith, A., & Cowper, D. (2005). Confronting an identity crisis – how to "brand" systems engineering. *Systems Engineering*, *8*(2), 164–186.

Fitzmaurice, E., & Richmond, J. (2017). An investigation of service providers' understanding, perspectives and implementations of the transdisciplinary model in early intervention settings for children with disabilities. *Internet Journal of Allied Health Sciences and Practice*, *15*(2).

Grootjans, J. (2010). White skin, black masks: a personal narrative on benevolent racism. In V. A. Brown, J. A. Harris, & J. Russel (Eds.), *Tackling wicked problems through the transdisciplinary imagination* (pp. 225–232). Earthscan.

Hammell, K. R. W., & Iwama, M. K. (2012). Well-being and occupational rights: an imperative for critical occupational therapy. *Scandinavian Journal of Occupational Therapy*, *19*(5), 385–394.

Iwama, M. K., Thomson, N. A., & Macdonald, R. M. (2009). The Kawa model: the power of culturally responsive occupational therapy. *Disability and Rehabilitation*, *31*(14), 1125–1135.

Koen, H., Roodt, H., & de Villiers, J. P. (2017). System-level causal modelling of widescale resource plundering: acting on the rhino poaching catastrophe. *Futures*, *93*, 102–114.

Lewis-Williams, J. D., & Pearce, D. G. (2004). *San spirituality: Roots, expression, and social consequences*. AltaMira Press.

MacLeod Schroeder, N.J. (2018). Rivers of doing, becoming, being, belonging: Exploring occupational therapist identity. [Doctor of Philosophy, University of Manitoba].https://mspace.lib.umanitoba.ca/xmlui/handle/1993/33290

McGregor, S. L. T. (2020). Transdisciplinarity and transpraxis. *Transdisciplinary Journal of Engineering & Science, 11.* https://doi.org/10.22545/2020/00134

Mobjörk, M. (2010). Consulting versus participatory transdisciplinarity: a refined classification of transdisciplinary research. *Futures, 42*(8), 866–873.

Montuori, A., & Donnelly, G. (2016). The creativity of culture and the culture of creativity research: the promise of integrative transdisciplinarity. In V. P. Glăveanu (Ed.), *The Palgrave handbook of creativity and culture research* (pp. 743–765). Palgrave Macmillan UK.

Morin, E. (2008). *On complexity.* Hampton Press.

Nagel, E., & Newman, J. R. (2001). *Gödel's proof (revised).* New York University Press.

Neuhauser, L. (2018). Practical and scientific foundations of transdisciplinary research and action. In D. Fam, L. Neuhauser, & P. Gibbs (Eds.), *Transdisciplinary theory, practice and education* (pp. 25–38). Springer.

Nicolescu, B. (2006). Transdisciplinarity: past, present and future. www.tercercongreso-mundialtransdisciplinariedad.mx/wp-content/uploads/2019/08/Transdisciplinarity-past-present-and-future.pdf

Nicolescu, B. (2010). Methodology of transdisciplinarity–levels of reality, logic of the included middle and complexity. *Transdisciplinary Journal of Engineering & Science, 1.* https://doi.org/10.22545/2010/0009

Nicolescu, B. (2014). Methodology of transdisciplinarity. *World Futures, 70*(3–4), 186–199.

Nicolescu, B. (2018). The transdisciplinary evolution of the university condition for sustainable development. In D. Fam, L. Neuhauser, & P. Gibbs (Eds.), *Transdisciplinary theory, practice and education* (pp. 73–81). Springer.

Roux, D. J., Nel, J. L., Cundill, G., O'Farrell, P., & Fabricius, C. (2017). Transdisciplinary research for systemic change: who to learn with, what to learn about and how to learn. *Sustainability Science, 12*(5), 711–726.

Ruwhiu, D., & Cathro, V. (2014). 'Eyes-wide-shut': insights from an indigenous research methodology. *Emergence: Complexity and Organization, 16*(4). https://journal.emergentpublications.com/Article/ae2ef77a-0b02-4a47-99a3-dfda00eb6a14/academic

Satterfield, J. M., Spring, B., Brownson, R. C., Mullen, E. J., Newhouse, R. P., Walker, B. B., & Whitlock, E. P. (2009). Toward a transdisciplinary model of evidence-based practice. *Milbank Quarterly, 87*(2), 368–390.

Stacey, R. D. (2001). *Complex responsive processes in organizations: Learning and knowledge creation.* Routledge.

Unruh, A. M. (2004). Reflections on: "So. . . What Do You Do?" Occupation and the construction of identity. *Canadian Journal of Occupational Therapy, 71*(5), 290–295.

Whyte, D. (2009). *The three marriages: Reimagining work, self and relationship.* Riverhead Books.

Woermann, M. (2013). *On the (im) possibility of business ethics: Critical complexity, deconstruction, and implications for understanding the ethics of business* (Vol. 37). Springer Science & Business Media.

Woermann, M., & Cilliers, P. (2012). The ethics of complexity and the complexity of ethics. *South African Journal of Philosophy, 31*(2), 447–463.

Young, K. (2019). Transdisciplinary Education Model: Embedding Occdupational Therapists into Specialised School Settings. University of Technology, Sydney. https://opus.lib.uts.edu.au/bitstream/10453/135551/1/Shire%20Schools%20-%20OT%20Project%20-%20Report%201%20FINAL.pdf

CHAPTER 9

Tools for Implementing the Five Finger Framework

Ideas, Activities, and Tips for Practice and Education Settings

Helen Jeffery[1] and Jan Hendrik Roodt[2]

[1]Principal Lecturer, School of Occupational Therapy, Te Pūkenga|Otago Polytechnic, New Zealand
[2]Advanced Academic Facilitator, Te Pūkenga, New Zealand

Frameworks provide a way of putting synthesized knowledge into practice – whether the "practice" be thinking or action. This chapter offers some tools and activity ideas that can be used by individuals or groups with the Five Finger Framework (FFF). The tools provide some structure to use of the framework in specific situations, and some creativity in how learners and practitioners might integrate it into their work. Most of the tools are suitable for learners in educational settings, novice practitioners, and experienced practitioners.

These tools may be used and adapted to fit your needs and context.

Professional Reasoning in Healthcare: Navigating Uncertainty Using the Five Finger Framework, First Edition.
Edited by Helen Jeffery, Linda Robertson, Jan Hendrik Roodt, and Susan Ryan.
© 2024 John Wiley & Sons Ltd. Published 2024 by John Wiley & Sons Ltd.

RESOURCE ONE

Template for Using the Five Finger Framework	
The decision I need to make is:	
Research and literature Put the question that guides your literature search, the references you select and a summary of key points here:	
Context and environment e.g., policy direction, resources, local culture, etc. Identify what you are guided to do by the context, what resources you have and what barriers that will affect your decision:	
Client insights – directly from the client/group and from multiple other sources. Identify the client's perspective and what you have learned from other sources. How can you best work in collaboration with this person/group at this time?	
Expertise of others – use peer experience and knowledge, expertise from internet resources. Note key learning that can influence your decision.	
Use of self – your own knowledge from experience, your attitudes and biases and values, what it is about you that is useful in making this decision. Also think about what you do not know, what you need to learn.	

RESOURCE TWO

Using the Five Finger Framework to Formulate a Case Presentation

Case presentations following this framework can be a useful way to:

- learn from and share learning from a specific practice example
- highlight enablers and barriers to service delivery
- influence the practice of peers and colleagues
- influence service development.

Introduction

Overview of reason for presentation (is this following assessment, a progress presentation, discharge, or reflection on how the whole process went, are you asking for input from the audience or simply presenting what happened?)

Client

- Overview of client (who was the client – individual/family/group/community?).
- Reason for referral or access to the service.
- Demographics.
- Relevant history.
- Ethnicity and culture, and influence this had on your decisions.
- Client's expertise – what did they bring to help you work out together what to do, and how did you ascertain this?
- Client's expectations from the service provided and how you ascertained this.

- Enablers to person-centered practice you identified – systems, resources, your approach, documentation, client's willingness to collaborate?
- Barriers to person-centered practice you identified – systems, resources, your approach, documentation, client's willingness to collaborate.
- Identify what you knew about people with similar health challenges and how you learned this (e.g., support groups, literature, previous clients, media).

Literature

- Describe the model of practice or approach you selected for intervention and justify.
- Refer to key research that provides evidence for decisions.
- Consider any barriers you had to implementing the research.
- Consider adaptations you may have made to the model or approach selected.
- Identify barriers and enablers to being able to access and use research and literature in the service.

Context and Environment

- Consider the barriers and enablers in your workplace regarding your practice with this client/group and describe their impact on decisions. Consider your access to resources (e.g., physical materials and equipment, spaces to work in, time, colleagues), workflow patterns (client pathways through the service, how work is allocated to staff, etc.).
- Identify the key protocols/guidelines and service practices that influenced your decisions.

- Describe the wider community context in which the client/group is situated and the influence this had on your work. Consider socio-economic situation, ethnicity, culture, geographical location. etc.

Expertise of Others

- Acknowledge the assistance you got from others in the workplace (e.g., peers, manager, supervisor) and identify the place they had in your decision making.
- Consider assistance from others in the wider community that you may have received – other services, groups, or individuals with expertise.
- Identify higher level expertise that might have influenced your work, if any – conference presentations, online videos or websites, formal professional development opportunities.

Self

- Reflect on your strengths, qualities, and skills – identify what you have within yourself that you demonstrated with this client/group. What

might others hear you say or see you do that portrays your way of working? What is it about who you are and how you operate that was helpful?
- Identify the role/s you took in the relationship – e.g., advocating, assisting, collaborating, teaching/instructing, supporting, empathizing, problem solving, hands-on therapy, assessing, providing feedback.
- What knowledge did you have that was useful in this instance?
- What were your knowledge gaps and what did or will you do about them?
- Reflecting on this experience, what has helped you develop or learn and what will you do with this new knowledge?

Summary

- Outcome for the client.
- Outcome for yourself (satisfaction, learning, goals).
- Potential outcome for the service – does this presentation alert you to any potential changes that could enhance the overall service provision?
- Recommendations.

RESOURCE THREE

Using the Five Finger Framework to Explore Research and Literature

Undertaking a critical review is an important task when determining the credibility of the research, but it is time consuming and requires an exacting set of skills. When time is limited and skills of critiquing research are constrained, it can be useful to follow guidelines that have a focus on the specific *context* of the research and its applicability in your situation, as much as its research *credibility*. The following questions can be usefully employed in situations where focus on utility is important. They are presented within the FFF.

Questions about a Published Research Article or a Textbook Summary

---

Myself

What relevant knowledge and experience do I have?
Can I link this to what I know and how I work?
To what degree is this relevant to me in my role?
Who is the information aimed at?
What are my beliefs about the value of these findings? What am I basing this on (e.g., personal beliefs and experiences, what you have read, what you have heard from others)?
Were there ethical issues that I believe were addressed or not considered?

Expertise of others

Who were the authors, were they key authorities on the subject, and how do you know this?
Have other experts in the topic paid attention to this study?
Is there evidence of consultation with key authorities?
Who has been referenced?
Are there other references that might be more helpful?

The client

Who were the participants?
How were participants selected/recruited?
What are the characteristics of the participants? How well does this correlate with your client group (e.g., age, gender, ethnicity)?
Where were the clients located (e.g., city, suburbs, rural districts, an institution)?
Did they have any input into the development or evaluation of the study?

The context

Where was the study located?
What similarities and differences exist between the research context and the scenario that is being considered (e.g., culture, staffing levels, expectations of management, resources)?
What impact did local/institutional policies and resources have on the intervention? (Could you do the same project in your setting?)

The decision being made

Overall: what decision have you made about the relevance/importance/value/validity of this study to inform your practice?
Rate out of five and provide justification.

RESOURCE FOUR

Activities to Stimulate Use of the Five Finger Framework with Learners

These resources form the basis of small group activities that are helpful for developing critical thinking and an awareness of the complexity integral to professional reasoning. Rich discussion and valuable teachable moments are likely to emerge as the learners justify their decisions and compare differences in the decisions for the same question. Good preparation will take some time but the same resources can be used multiple time and in a variety of ways with the same group or with different groups.

Bingo	

Your preparation	• Write/prepare the resources that are described on the cards. This will take time – you can adapt the suggestions (table 1) to create a good fit with the learner's situation.
	• Prepare the brief scenario (or use the one provided).
	• Prepare practice questions or descriptions of a decision to be made that links with the scenario and your profession. Ensure the decision (even if complex) can be articulated simply—an **either/or** format is ideal.
	• Make the boards, each 5 squares × 5 squares. As many boards as you need for the size of the group.
	• Have five cards of each of five colors. The colors represent the fingers on the Five Finger Framework.
	  • Gray = myself
	  • Green = expertise of others
	  • Orange = client
	  • Blue = context and environment
	  • White = research and literature
	• On one side of the card is the description of the resource (see table 1).
	• On the other side of each card is a number between 1 and 25 (random, ensure the numbers are not on the same card for each board).
	• Have bingo numbers to select during the game – only numbers 1–25 required.

Playing the game	• Organize the learners into small groups (two or more in each group). • One board is provided to each group, along with a complete set of cards. The group lays the cards on the board randomly, with the number side up. • Have a caller – when each number is called, the group can turn its card over and request its resource. • After each number, the group has time to read/view its resource and make its provisional decision. You may choose to have the group share its decision with the whole group, but not to discuss or justify yet. • After five numbers are drawn, the group makes its final decision and shares with the whole group what its decision is and how they justify it. • Discuss as a group.

(Continued)

(Continued)

Auction	
Your preparation	• Write/prepare the resources that are described on the cards. This will take time – you can adapt the suggestions (table 1) to create a good fit with the learner's situation. • Prepare the brief scenario (or use the one provided). • Prepare practice questions or descriptions of a decision to be made that links with the scenario and your profession. Ensure the decision (even if complex) can be articulated simply—an **either/or** format is ideal. • Have Monopoly® money or tokens available.
Playing the game	• Have learners work in small groups. • Ensure they understand what colored card represents which finger on the framework. • As the auctioneer, select a card and present it for sale. The card and associated resource go to the highest bidder. • Keep auctioning cards; once each group has at least one card, pause the auction. • Set a timeframe for learners to come to their decision. • Have each group justify its decision. Discuss as a group. • Play another round if there is time.

The scenario presented relates to one of the chapters in this text. Facilitating the activity session and then providing the chapter as follow-up reading will strengthen learners' understanding, even if the scenario in the chapter is of a person from a different profession from yours. You can develop other scenarios and boards that relate to the other chapters in the book and use in the same way. Equally, you can develop a scenario that is a good fit for your profession or workplace.

Scenario for the Learners

Marty is a 37-year-old manager of a large inner-city business. He sustained trauma to his neck in a car accident which led to a cerebral vascular accident (CVA) with damage to the Broca's area. He has associated Broca's aphasia; although able to string some sentences together, he has considerable difficulty with word finding. He also has some right-sided weakness affecting his overall function.

Brief notes on Marty's home situation including Asian ethnicity, family, employment situation, financial security. etc.	**Myself** The strengths and qualities you have, your beliefs and your style of working. What do you have within you that will influence this decision?	Copy of an initial assessment appropriate for the service that has been completed about Marty.	Written overview of a relationship model or style of therapeutic interviewing.	Notes from an education session you attended about cross-cultural practice in your healthcare setting.
You have two years' experience working with people who have had a stroke, notes on specific practices or approaches in which you have developed expertise.	Video of a young person who has experienced a stroke.	Notes from a meeting with your manager where parameters for time and facility resources are outlined.	Copy of a report about Marty's job, including job type, the physical and cognitive demands, and the social environment at his workplace.	Copy of national stroke guidelines.
Overview of the community services available for Marty that he might benefit from.	Notes on a conversation with a colleague about how to manage to work effectively within the resources available.	Copy of notes following a conversation with Marty's extended family and the role they plan to have in his care.	Notes from your attendance at a stroke support group – what you discovered that might be helpful with your decision.	Copy of standard service provision protocols including time frames, discharge planning, and therapist resources.
Progress report from a practitioner of another profession who is also working with Marty.	Health condition analysis on stroke using International Classification of Function.	Notes from a cultural supervision session where you talk through the cultural differences in healthcare beliefs between you and the client.	Session notes following a conversation you have with Marty about his family's involvement and how he envisions his future.	A written reflection triggered by discovering that a team member from another profession had a different view of progress.
Copy of an article exploring cross-cultural healthcare, particularly collectivist and individualist.	Notes from a team meeting where you presented your work with Marty and received feedback.	Copy of an article outlining best practice in stroke rehabilitation for your profession.	Video of presentation on best practice stroke rehabilitation in your profession.	Copy of the goals Marty has set with you.

Gathering the Evidence Using the Five Finger Framework

Research and Literature	Context and Environment	Client	Expertise of Others	Myself
Where will I find this evidence?	**Where will I find this evidence?**	**Where will I find this evidence?**	**Where will I find this evidence?**	**Where w.ill I find this evidence?**
• Research publications • Gray literature • Literature summaries – systematic reviews, scoping reviews • Theory (profession specific) • Textbooks • Conference presentations • Internet resources	• Policy, protocols and guidelines • Workplace practices • Legislation • Service resources • Community resources • Other services in the community	• Clients and family/ community • Client support groups • Websites • Literature specific to the client population	• Other practitioners • Opinion pieces • Online resources • Professional magazines • Books • Conference presentations • Supervisors and managers	• Reflections • Conversations • Insights • Feedback from others – clients, peers, supervisor, manager • Feedback from others who know me well
Questions that I might ask	**Questions that I might ask**	**Questions that I might ask**	**Questions that I might ask**	**Questions that I might ask**
• What is the research evidence base for this decision, how can the research and literature help me work out what to do and how to do it?	• How do I do things here, in this place, and what can help me ascertain this?	• What is the clients' perspective and situation, how can I best ascertain this and collaborate with them to good effect?	• Who can help me with this decision, and how best can I access their expertise?	• What is familiar about this, what do I already know, what do I need to know and how can I find it out, how can I make best use of myself in this situation?

- What research evidence is available to help me?
- What is considered best practice?
- Is there a model or framework appropriate in this situation?
- What assessments can best help identify the issue?
- What outcomes are relevant/acceptable?
- What theoretical frameworks can help me to understand this issue?

- What national policies and frameworks are relevant?
- What local protocols and guidelines are relevant?
- How do I implement the guidelines in this service?
- Team and service cultural influences.
- Community cultural influences.
- What cultural issues are likely to impact on practice?
- What pressures are affecting this situation?
- What risks need to be considered?
- Who else is working with this client?
- What resources are available?

- Who is the client and what is their main concern?
- What outcomes are they expecting?
- What support is available to them?
- What is their understanding of their health condition?
- What are their strengths?
- What are their values/customs?
- What is the client's experience of this and what expertise do they hold?
- What can be learned about the client's situation through the internet, local support groups, etc.?

- What is usually done in this setting (i.e., the interventions)?
- What is usually done by this profession?
- What are the parameters that are used to judge best practice?
- Why is this considered to be successful?
- What assessments are relevant?
- What team members are involved in decision making?
- What does an expert expect for this situation?

- What experiences and knowledge do you have that will be helpful here?
- What kind of communicator are you?
- What values and beliefs guide your practice?
- How strong/committed are you in your ethical practice journey?
- What are your strengths?
- How vulnerable are you in this situation?
- What kind of reasoning are you using?

RESOURCE SIX

Stimulating Intentional Reflection

Reflection facilitates learning from experiences – it is where you make meaning from the experience that is a good fit with who you are and what you know. Reflection *in* action refers to reflective processes in the moment (while engaged in a task); reflection *on* action refers to looking back to an event once it is finished.

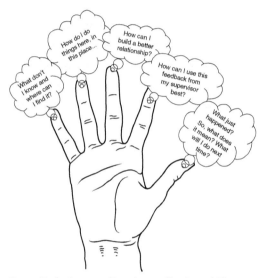

Some Techniques to Develop Reflection Skills and Habits

- **Keep a brief diary**. At the end of each day, jot down some sentences. This may provide you with material that you want to explore further, e.g., in supervision, help you identify themes that are a strength for you and themes that point to changes you need to make, and help you recognize learning moments. For structure, select from the following ideas or write whatever comes to mind. Look back on what you have written occasionally; if there are themes, this might be where you need to focus a

more formal reflection. Remember, if you keep it short (2–4 sentences), it is more likely to become a daily habit. These questions might also be helpful in group supervision to get conversation going.

- What brought satisfaction or joy in my work today? AND what brought anxiety or frustration or another uncomfortable feeling in my work today?
- A moment I felt on top of my game today AND a moment I felt out of my depth today.
- Something helpful from someone else today AND something unhelpful from someone else today.
- Something I learned today AND something I now know I need to learn.
- An "ah-ha!" moment from today and an "oh no!" moment from today.
- A surprise from today AND a disappointment from today.
- Something I am grateful for from today AND something I feel resentful about from today.
- What struck me about today?
- Who do I look forward to seeing again (and why) AND who am I not looking forward to seeing again (and why)?
- Some feedback I got today that is helpful AND what I will do about it.
- Something I read today that struck me AND why.
- A dilemma from today AND one thing I will do to work toward addressing it.
- A question from today AND an answer from today.
- **Have objects and pictures to trigger reflection**. Keep them on your desk, on a shelf or in a drawer or

a box. This is helpful when reflecting alone, in a group such as team development meetings or peer supervision, or with your supervisor or supervisee. Sometimes the metaphor that forms when holding the object or pictures of objects helps with clarity of understanding or expressing what is happening. You might choose to intentionally select a particular object/picture, or to select randomly. Some ideas are given below.

- A stick: what has stuck with me about this?
- A shell ("What shall I do about this"): triggers goal setting.
- A magnifying glass: what do I need to explore in much more depth?
- A cup: what is filling my cup and what is emptying it?
- A blossom or flower: what is blossoming in me, how do I think I am developing as a practitioner?
- A picture of an ear: something I have heard that is helpful and/or challenging.
- Picture of a hare and tortoise: what do I rush through and what do I take my time over (and why)?
- Calendar page: what's a good day of the week for me (and why) AND what's not a good day of the week for me (and why)?
- A leaf: what do I need to leave behind?
- A rock: may represent something that is hard for you right now, or something that is great – it "rocks"!
- A mirror: when I look at myself as a health practitioner, I see. . . or when I reflect on this situation, I see. . .
- A book: something I am reading about that is helpful.
- A camera: a powerful moment/experience I have captured.
- A magic wand: I wish . . .

- **Find a reflection model that resonates with you**. Most of them are process orientated – experiment with different ways of going through the process to find out what suits you best. It might be thinking or talking (with another or in a group), writing, mind-mapping or drawing. Honesty is important to get genuine depth. Remember, it is important that reflection helps you reinforce good practice and make changes to enhance practice. The "what" to reflect on may be triggered by some of the ideas above. Often it is obvious – an uncomfortable feeling has arisen in you and is telling you to think about what caused it and how to resolve it.
- **Link reflective thoughts to the FFF**. By regularly identifying which finger/s you are spending time on, you will start to identify your learning needs or practice/service changes that would be helpful; for example, not having enough time in sessions for thorough client education might result in the service sourcing or developing education resources for clients.
- **Present at a case conference**. Structuring the presentation on what happened throughout your time with the client because of your decisions based on each of the fingers, and finishing with a discussion on what worked well and what could have been done differently will help the thumb grow and give you material to reflect on further (see case presentation template above).

RESOURCE SEVEN

Teaching Sessions for Five Finger Framework

Preparation

The preparation might take some time but once done, it can be used in different ways with different learners. These ideas will work in the classroom and in practice settings.

Write a case scenario that includes triggers for further exploration of features related to each finger. You can use the example below, or modify it, or develop your own. You may choose to use the chapters in this text to base your scenario on (adapt the setting and client to meet parameters of your profession and learner group) and follow up with providing the chapter as adjunctive reading.

Formulate a question that requires a decision from the practitioner that fits the scenario for the learners to work on. Formulate any question that fits your profession and learner needs; some ideas to get you started are given below.

- You have just completed the initial assessment. What other information do you require and how will you access it? (Develop and provide a copy of an initial assessment.)
- You need to present the case to the team and request more time/resources. What information will you include and why?
- You have decided to do a session with the client that is educational so that they can learn more about the health condition. What resources will you use to develop the plan, where and when and how will you do it?
- There is a peak in referrals to your service and you need to reduce the

amount of time each week you can spend with the client. What can you do to ensure they are still getting a good service and their needs are being met?

Develop finger-specific resources that are in line with the scenario. These are any resources that will help the group delve deeper but that are not generic – learners can source generic resources themselves. They might be linked to the question. An example for each finger is provided below.

- Work context and environment parameters – workflow, resources available (materials, equipment, time, vehicle access, spaces to work in) (context and environment finger).
- A particular intervention/approach/model that is to be used (literature finger).
- Some detail about the client situation such as their relationship with the practitioner, their social context, a stressor they have now, their past history in health services. Make sure it builds on what is in the scenario – something surprising and difficult will stimulate the learners (client finger).
- The access the practitioner has to supervision and knowledgeable others in the service – be specific so it fits with the scenario (expertise of others finger).
- A written reflection that covers workload pressures and some of the challenges the practitioner is facing (thumb).

The Session

Split into small groups and allocate each small group a finger to work on. Ensure they have the resources needed – the scenario, their finger-specific resource, devices to access internet and databases, copy of this text, etc. Instructions for the learners are as follows.

- Read the scenario and identify the information in it that fits with your finger. Remember some points will fit with more than one finger – that is OK.
- Read the adjunctive notes you have that pertain to your finger, and use the internet and your own knowledge and resources to develop a fuller picture of the scenario.
- Consider the question/decision point you have been provided.
- Research, think together as a group, and decide what to do from the perspective of the finger you are working on.
- Prepare a presentation for the whole group (two minutes) where you declare your decision and your rationale for it.

Have each group present, and then facilitate discussion as a whole group about the decision and the complexity behind it. Formulate a clear decision as a whole group.

Adaptations for Multiple Sessions

- Repeat with same scenario and different decision points/questions; maybe move through the therapeutic process – initial assessment, goal setting, intervention/practice decisions, moving on.
- Same session and scenario but add something dramatic to the scenario so the situation is very different for the client.
- Have the group work in small subgroups but on the same finger; repeat the session plan for each finger.
- Develop a poster as a group that portrays the value of that finger in professional decision making.

- Repeat with different scenarios – if using this text, you may choose to base the scenarios on the ones presented here (adapt so they fit with your context).
- Repeat but have each small group work with every finger; the whole-group discussion at the end will compare the decisions made by each group and their rationale.
- Same scenario and process but have an **either/or** question (e.g., for this older person you are working with, will you recommend she remains at home or is supported into a care facility?). Have students form two teams and allocate an answer to each team. After they are prepared, set up a debate to justify how they got to the decision provided for them using information from each finger.

Educational Formative or Summative Assessment Ideas

- **Poster presentations** (individual or small group) on the finger or the whole framework.
- **Written assignment** on the scenario covered in class, or different scenario.
- **Oral assessment** based on one of the scenarios you have developed (see oral assessment question ideas in this chapter).
- **Written reflection** from fieldwork education experience where the client is described, a decision point is evident (this might be as simple as: what will I do the next time I see the client and why?) and use of each of the fingers is evident.
- **Case presentation** based on a client from fieldwork education experience (see case presentation template above for ideas).

RESOURCE EIGHT

Using the Five Finger Framework as a Supervisor

- Have a picture of the hand on a piece of paper and encourage the supervisee to touch base with each finger as they describe a practice situation.
- Use mind-mapping on the drawing of the hand to facilitate links between the fingers, the thumb, and the situation being described.
- Ensure that the supervisee focuses on each finger in turn and does not tend to focus on just one.
- Identify a particular finger for the supervisee to expand on, to enable deeper reasoning.
- Help the supervisee identify skills, knowledge, and qualities they have through a strengths-based focus on the thumb.
- Have the supervisee identify an insight, learning or knowledge gap at the end of supervision for them to set a professional development goal.
- Have the supervisee identify resources or system changes that would enable or enhance the use of all the fingers in the framework.
- Share your own knowledge or advise when it seems appropriate.
- Recommend learning opportunities and resources related to each finger (over time); ensure your focus covers the breadth of the framework.
- Orientate the supervisee to resources in the service or community they may not be aware of.

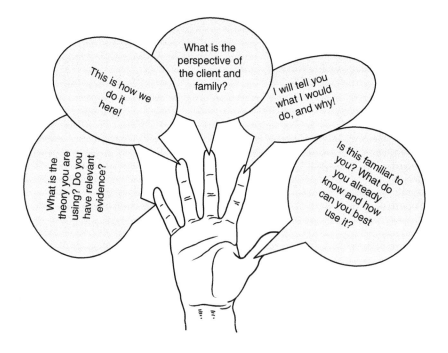

RESOURCE NINE

Using the Five Finger Framework to Structure a Client- or Scenario-based Oral Assessment or Review

These questions will help the learner think both broadly and deeply about the given scenario.

Source of Evidence	Questions that Might be Helpful
Research and literature finger	• What is the main body of literature that you have found most useful for you with this scenario, and why is that? • Can you talk a bit about how the literature has helped you with your decisions? • Is there anything about what you discovered in the research literature that is difficult for you to consider or use in this situation? • How might you contextualize the research literature, so it is a better fit for your workplace?
Environment/ context finger	• What are some of the contextual features of the work environment that you have had to consider? • In what ways do you think your work environment in this scenario has influenced your decisions with this client? • What are some of the cultural factors related to the local environment (social and/or physical environments) that you have had to consider here? How has this influenced your decisions?
Client finger	• We know that it is important to have the client central to our decisions – what are some things that you have considered that illustrates client-centeredness? • Tell me a little bit about how what you know about the client as a person has influenced your decisions here? • What can you do in this instance to better understand the client's perspective? • Is there anything you can do to better understand what the client's experience might be here other than asking the client more questions?
Expertise of others finger	• Who are the other people in your work environment that you might go to for help or information? • You have talked about the research literature that you have read; are there any other ways in which you have used the voice of other people who have expertise in this area?
Use of self	• In terms of this client and situation, what is one thing that you might want to take to supervision and why might you do this? • What is something about you as a person that would be helpful in this situation with this client? • Thinking about therapeutic use of self, what is one thing someone might see you do or hear you say that is intentional use of self? • You have spent a lot of time and energy preparing for this viva – how do you think it has helped you become better prepared for practice? • Now that you have done this piece of work, what are a couple of things about your knowledge and skills that you think need more work? • What is a new piece of learning that really stands out for you having completed this course or worked with this person?

RESOURCE TEN

Developing Transdisciplinary Practice

1. Consider a recent case study. Using your current model of practice, map the role that each finger might or might not play in the development of the intervention. Reflect in a critical manner on the adequacy of the outcome and consider to what extent, if at all, use of the FFF would have altered the outcome.

2. Using the same case study, change the client cultural/religious/social position to represent a likely future client. Now apply the FFF to devise an intervention that would follow the transdisciplinary approach and values described in chapter eight. Critically reflect on this anticipatory exercise as a sense-making event.

3. Repeat (2) in a group setting where the group members offer ideas on post-it notes pasted on six areas on a wall, named after the five fingers and their descriptions, and the sixth is named "Intervention." Cluster ideas and discuss the emerging patterns.

Tips

- Think about "levels of reality." Consider using the word "AND" rather than the word "OR" when considering ideas, especially when thinking about solutions.

- Think about the interaction of different combinations of the "fingers": the thumb in interaction with the index finger and the middle finger while also "talking" to the fourth finger. Assign people to represent these fingers and role-play the process of collaborative practice.

- Start a practice team library for paradigms other than the western world view and invite speakers from diverse cultural backgrounds to learning and development days or sessions.

Index

Professional Reasoning in Healthcare: Navigating Uncertainty Using the Five Finger Framework, First Edition.
Edited by Helen Jeffery, Linda Robertson, Jan Hendrik Roodt, and Susan Ryan.
© 2024 John Wiley & Sons Ltd. Published 2024 by John Wiley & Sons Ltd.